MOVEMENT + MUSIC = MEDICINE

Fight Alzheimer's, Dementia & Parkinson's

Jem Spectar

Table of Contents

Reviews of Movement + Music = Medicine

"This well-researched book with intriguing and insightful anecdotes makes a substantial contribution towards understanding how movement, particularly dance, may help slow the course of Alzheimer's and Parkinson's diseases. The book is especially relevant and timely, given the alarming increase in the two diseases - medical conditions often associated with aging but highly variable between patients. *Movement + Music = Medicine* is highly recommended for a general audience seeking to learn more about neurological disorders and how lifestyle changes, particularly movement, exercise, and dance, may make a difference."
Arthur S. Levine, M.D. Executive Director, University of Pittsburgh Brain Institute, Professor of Medicine, Molecular Genetics, and Neurobiology. Senior Vice Chancellor Emeritus, Health Sciences, Dean Emeritus, School of Medicine, University of Pittsburgh.

"Dr. Spectar has created a masterpiece combining the history of dance across culture and time and the evidence to support brain health and combatting neurodegenerative disease. He weaves throughout the book, vivid imagery of lively dancers from ancient Greece to the nursing home down the road. I am convinced, I will now be prescribing dance to my patients, for lasting limberness of the brain and the body."
Mylynda B. Massart, M.D., Ph.D., Physician and co-director, Clinical and Translational Science Institute, University of Pittsburgh.

"I have never seen a compilation of science and humanities so beautifully intertwined—like a dance in and of itself! ... Through the lens of health and healing, Dr. Jem Spectar masterfully crafts the interrelationship between science and art as supported by a vast collection of empirical data, multicultural applications, and personal narratives that argue for the critical need of dance and movement to sustain a healthy society... Movement + Music = Medicine provides a substantial contribution to the growing field of Medical Humanities within medical schools, graduate studies, residency programs, public health departments, and, of course, dance... [This] book is phenomenal!" **Susan Wieczorek, Ph.D.**, Associate Professor of Communications; a thought leader in the emerging field of Medical Humanities, University of Pittsburgh Johnstown.

"As caregiver for a spouse struggling with late-stage Alzheimer's Disease, reading this enormously resourceful book makes me wonder what life for us might be like today if the book had been available earlier in our journey. Upon receiving the diagnosis four years ago, we explored a wide range of books and other publications for answers to questions about what Alzheimer's Disease is, why it afflicts people, and what cures or treatments were available. While exercise and physical activity were underscored repeatedly in the readings as potentially beneficial supplements to medication, nowhere was the combination of music and dance even intimated as a therapeutic resource for delaying the onset of Alzheimer's Disease and its accompanying neurological, physiological, and psychological impairments. Dr. Spectar's book appears to fill a void in therapeutic resources for Alzheimer's Disease patients and caregivers...
I highly recommend this book for anyone who suspects a neurological disease may become an issue in their family.

It's a must read for newly diagnosed patients with a neurological disease and for family members caring for patients who are advancing through various stages of the diseases." **Livy – a caregiver.**

*****

Why Movement + Music = Medicine? Why Now? I believe we are all increasingly at grave risk for neurological disorders, including Alzheimer's, dementia, and Parkinson's - diseases that inflict a staggering toll on the afflicted and their loved ones. Most troubling, current pharmacological interventions are not cures and do not often provide needed relief. This book will inform and empower you to develop a plan of action to help you or your loved one fight against Alzheimer's, Parkinson's, and other neurological disorders. Informed by relevant research, this book shows that movement or exercise, particularly when combined with music, has a powerful impact on brain health. The scientific research is also illuminated and amplified by the lived experiences of people whose stories reveal how movement, exercise, and dance therapy are giving them an edge in the struggle against neurological disorders. *Movement + Music = Medicine* will increase your knowledge about the medicinal impact of rhythmic movement and give you greater confidence to make decisions that can improve your brain health.

About the Author

Jem Spectar, PhD, JD, MBA, MA, MAP, is the President of the University of Pittsburgh at Johnstown. Forthcoming books include: We Dance for Light: Lifestyle Medicine for Depression, Anxiety & Stress and Rx MED: Preventive Medicine for Heart Disease, Cancer and Diabetes & Healthy Aging.

I. Understanding Alzheimer's, Dementia & Parkinson's

The "Color Sisters," Diann White and Jakki Brown, rule the dance floor at the University of Pennsylvania's weekly dance program for older adults in the City of Brotherly and Sisterly Love, Philadelphia.[1] The colorful moniker, derived from their last names, might as well be a vivid description of their spirited dancing to the upbeat music and choreography of David Earley and Selena Williams, a husband and wife team of dance instructors hired by the university.[2] The Brown-White duo, who met and bonded in the course of the program, is described as "the life of the class." Passionate about music and dancing, they are typically the first on the dance floor and could be seen moving to the beat until the very end of the last dance.[3] Started by Dr. Terri Lipman of U Penn Nursing in 2013, Dance for Health is run by Penn Memory Center (PMC) to promote healthy lifestyles, improve brain health, and reduce the prevalence of neurodegenerative diseases like dementia and Alzheimer's.[4] Designed for older adults, including some participants who have cognitive impairments, the weekly dance program is open to people with varying levels of dancing skills.[5] Activities are structured so everyone could join in with fun choreographic moves such as line dances that combine a series of simple steps with movements uniquely tailored to the varying needs of older adults.[6] A major additional benefit of the program is the opportunity to meet other people, develop friendships, and increase participants' social connectedness.[7] The program also includes monthly intergenerational health promotion activities involving students from area high schools.[8] Students from the University of Pennsylvania Master's in Public Health (MPH) also engage with program participants during classes and keep track of the pedometers that track participants' steps. [9]

Dance for Health participants complete surveys about their well-being and satisfaction with their everyday lives at the beginning and end of each session; feedback from community members has been very positive.[10] Mildred Johnson, a retiree, who joined the program over eight years ago, has been a regular attendee and participant in the weekly dance classes. [11] Embracing the program's core messaging about healthy lifestyles and healthy aging over the longer term, Ms. Johnson declared: "I need this ... I want to be independent." Jakki Brown, one half of the Color Sisters, touts the program's goal of promoting social connectedness, stating, "I prefer physical activity with people... With people, I am more prone to do it. It's difficult to do physical activity by myself."[12]   Danielle Kennedy, then an MPH student interning at the program, was, at first, "unsure" about participating in the dance classes and was concerned because she had not had any prior line dancing class lessons.[13] However, after her initial reluctance, she was transformed into an eager participant who found herself looking forward to the weekly dance session and the opportunity it provided to strengthen her relationships with other people.[14] As Ms. Kennedy wrote in a follow-up reflection paper, dancing together with the seniors and others from the community "felt natural," and the experience helped her "connect with them."[15]   She also discovered that the community participants "enjoyed the social aspect of the program," and she was "able to witness firsthand how social dance can bring [people] joy and health." [16] Participants told her they were grateful for the program because Dance for Health "provided them with a break from their usual routine and a chance to connect with others."[17] Many participants brought friends or family members to class, while others formed new friendships and bonded over shared experiences.[18]

Dance? You wonder. The University of Pennsylvania, one of the world's greatest institutions, is running several weekly dance programs for seniors from its surrounding communities - to promote brain health. Why do rhythmic movement and dance help prevent, delay, or help 'manage' neurodegenerative disorders such as dementia and Alzheimer's Disease and Parkinson's Disease?[19] Before returning to this central question, it is, first of all, helpful to get a better understanding of the nature and etiology of these disorders and the limits of current pharmacological therapies.

*****

Dementia is a brain disease generally caused by a

perturbation of several higher cortical functions

resulting in memory loss or amnesia and other

significant cognitive changes that seriously impair

thinking, reasoning, communication, comprehension,

learning capacity, and judgment.[20]   Persons with

dementia also have difficulty navigating complexity,

problem-solving, planning, organizing, and coordinating

functions, and they often experience confusion, mood

swings, and disorientation.[21]   Forms of dementia

include Alzheimer's disease (about 60- 80 of dementia

cases), vascular dementia caused by high blood

pressure, alcohol-related dementia, Parkinson's

dementia, frontotemporal dementia, and various

dementia-like memory issues caused by several medical conditions.[22] Primary risk factors for dementia include advanced age as well as environmental, lifestyle, and genetic factors such as the common genetic polymorphism, the apolipoprotein E (APOE) e4 allele. [23] Other associated risk factors for advanced dementia may include head injury, depression, vascular disease, smoking, high blood pressure, high cholesterol and lower levels of educational attainment.[24]

Alzheimer's, the most common form of dementia, alters the brain by precipitating its atrophy, diminishing healthy cells and contributing to the development of defective cells characterized by beta-amyloid plaques and neurofibrillary or tau tangles.[25] The plaques are sticky clumps of proteins that build up between nerve cells while tangles are twisted fibers in the cells preventing movement of nutrients and information within the cell. [26] The increase in flawed cells with plaques and tangles injures surrounding healthy brain cells and causes their death, reducing the production of neurotransmitters and furthering brain shrinkage - a vicious self-reinforcing loop. [27] Researchers have determined a key risk factor is possessing one form of the apolipoprotein E (APOE) gene on chromosome 19 (which comes in several different forms or alleles), particularly APOE-4.[28]

Beyond genetics, scientists think a combination of environmental and lifestyle factors may be responsible for the onset of Alzheimer's and its progression.[29] Researchers theorize Alzheimer's is the product of a mix of age-related factors including shrinkage of the brain, inflammation, the production of free radicals or unstable molecules, the collapse of energy production inside cells, and increasingly sedentary behavior.[30] It is thought that sedentary behaviors among older adults may impact neurobiological processes, including reducing neurogenesis, synaptic plasticity, and BDNF production, while increasing inflammation and elevating risk of vascular disease.[31] Researchers are also exploring associations between cognitive decline and heart disease, stroke, high blood pressure, obesity, depression, and diabetes, as well as the extent to which diminishing the risk factors for these conditions lessens the risk of Alzheimer's.[32] For example, according to a long-term observational study published in *Diabetologia*, higher blood sugar levels may be linked to cognitive and executive function decline and memory loss.[33] After tracking 5,189 people for over a decade, researchers concluded that those with high blood sugar experienced a more rapid rate of neurodegenerative decline than those with normal blood sugar, even if they were merely pre-diabetic.[34] Study co-author Wuxiang

Xie at the Peking University Health Science Center remarked that while the underlying cause is unclear, vascular complications linked to diabetes could partially account for the subsequent memory loss. [35] The efficient utilization of glucose in the brain is seen as a key to effective thinking, memory, and learning, especially because the brain is a high-energy customer, consuming 50% of the body's sugar. [36] Just as too much glucose in the brain can result in cognitive deficiencies, a shortage of glucose in the brain also results in diminished production of neurotransmitters, and a breakdown of inter-neuronal communications.[37] Hypoglycemia, a potential complication of diabetes, also deprives the brain of energy and contributes to poor cognitive functioning.[38]

Furthermore, clinical depression, afflicting 5 percent of adults aged 65, may be a significant contributor to the rising cases of Alzheimer's and dementia among older persons.[39] A study published in the *British Journal of Psychiatry* by Meryl Butters and her colleagues at the Pitt School of Medicine concluded that late-life depression is linked to a significant risk of all-cause dementia.[40] After a meta-analysis consisting of 23 studies, the researchers concluded **36 of every 50 older adults with late-life depression could eventually develop vascular dementia, and 31 of every 50 seniors with a history of depression could develop Alzheimer's.**[41] The researchers suggest a 10 percent reduction in depression could prevent 68,000 cases of dementia annually.[42] It is thought that the link between depression and dementia/Alzheimer's may be high levels of the stress hormone cortisol, a typical occurrence in depressed persons.[43] Cortisol is thought to have a toxic effect on the hippocampus, possibly even contributing to its shrinkage and thereby compromising the storage of long-term memories. [44] For example, in an article published in *Aging Mental Health*, Kathryn Sawyer and her colleagues found evidence linking depression to a decrease in right hippocampal volume and also a connection between hippocampal volume and subsequent cognitive decline; a decrease in left and right hippocampal volume predicted decrease in the Mini Mental State Examination (MMSE) within 4 years.[45] The MMSE is typically used to develop an "objective measure of global cognitive functioning" in five areas - orientation, registration, attention and calculation, recall, and language; MMSE scores range from 0 – 30 with scores below 25 "generally indicative of cognitive impairment."[46] Researchers think depression may also fuel chronic inflammation which injures blood vessels and obstructs blood flow in the brain, fueling the decline of neural networks and increasing the risk of dementia.[47] Other researchers are also focusing on potential connections between poor sleep habits and rising dementia. [48] Sleepless in Seattle was a great movie, but sleeplessness anywhere is bad for brain health. Deep sleep enables the body to release hormones designed to repair cells and build tissue in the body and brain.[49] Some researchers have found a connection between insufficient sleep and the gradual accumulation of the insidious plaques and tangles in the brain that cause dementia and Alzheimer's. [50]

There are no known cures for dementia and Alzheimer's. Current treatments strive to control associated conditions or symptoms such as depression, anxiety, agitation, delusions, hallucinations, and related behavioral issues.[51] Treatments based on cholinesterase inhibitors aim at boosting the performance of brain chemicals that transmit information from one brain cell to another but do nothing to stop the underlying neurodegenerative decline and the continuous death of brain cells.[52] Given the very serious side effects of current drug interventions for dementia and Alzheimer's, experts often recommend initial non-drug-related psychosocial interventions as the first step to manage associated behavioral problems.[53] It is also recommended that interventions be initially aimed at identifying and treating the underlying physical, psychological or environmental causes.[54] Meanwhile, some are expressing alarm about the seeming over-reliance on antipsychotics to pacify dementia patients and the ensuing health damage. [55] In an article published in the British Medical Journal in 2015, Peter Gøtzsche and his colleagues argue that the benefit of these drugs are "minimal" relative to the harm they cause, arguing that up to 500,000 people over 65 in the West die annually as a result of the use of these psychiatric drugs.[56] For example, haloperidol and risperidone, two antipsychotic medications prescribed to lessen agitation and anxiety among dementia patients, have also been associated with a higher risk of death.[57]

Progress on new drug development has been slow, although some current developments are raising hopes. Recently, Biogen announced it is seeking regulatory approval for a drug called Aducanumab that will purportedly be the first therapy that could actually slow Alzheimer's disease by targeting and clearing away the toxic amyloid plaques.[58] Meanwhile, Chinese authorities have conditionally approved a new seaweed-based drug called Oligomannate for use in the treatment of mild to moderate Alzheimer's.[59] The team that developed the drug at the Shanghai Institute of Materia Medica was reportedly inspired by the relatively low incidence of Alzheimer's among people who eat seaweed regularly.[60] Other researchers are seeking to develop drugs to increase brain-derived neurotrophic factor or BDNF levels in the brain in a bid to trigger adult hippocampal neurogenesis or nerve cell growth and thereby restore brain functioning.[61] BDNF produces a rich environment where neurons thrive and forge new interconnections between cells, resulting in greater synaptic density.[62] Meanwhile, researchers at the University of Pennsylvania have achieved important breakthroughs in the science of triggering memory and recall by way of implanted electrodes and targeted electrical pulses in the brain.[63] Similarly, in April 2019, scientists reported that a new noninvasive approach called Transcranial Alternating Current Stimulation (TACS) could fix memory deficits by synchronizing and tuning neural circuits in certain areas in the frontal and temporal cortex affected by age-related decline.[64] This approach mimics and builds on the way brainwaves, known as theta waves, activate working memory by synchronizing neural circuits to one another.[65] The TACs reportedly emulate the way memory works across the brain, simulating the moves of an orchestra conductor, coordinating diverse musicians - synchronizing, harmonizing and fine-tuning them. [66]

Researchers are also exploring the possibility of interventions involving the hormone, klotho. Named after the capricious deity that spun ancient fates, klotho is normally produced by the kidneys and in the cells lining the brain's fluid-filled ventricles.[67] While plentiful in our blood at birth, the supply diminishes with aging, especially among those suffering from neurodegenerative disorders.[68] For example, researchers have observed that klotho is severely depleted among those afflicted with diseases such as Alzheimer's, dementia, and Parkinson's as well as those suffering from chronic stress and burnout.[69] In an article published in *Neurology*, researchers suggest klotho pathways might prevent the harmful impacts of APOE4 in aging and disease, and potentially changing APOE4-related variances in disease pathology.[70] The study effectively linked klotho with "attenuation of a key pathogenic protein and biomarker of neurodegenerative disease," suggesting it provides resilience to APOE4-linked pathways with regard to the onset of Alzheimer's.[71] Study co-author Dena Dubal suggests klotho revitalizes the aging brain by stimulating its electrical connections, perhaps by increasing strength in electrical signals going from cell to cell in the hippocampus.[72] Following an experiment that injected Klotho into mice, researchers observed that klotho appeared to rejuvenate even mice that showed signs of cognitive decline akin to the neurodegeneration typically associated with dementia,

Alzheimer's, Parkinson's, and multiple sclerosis.[73] In addition, the extra klotho turbo-charged the brains of healthy mice, boosting their resilience and longevity as well as their cognitive capacity with regard to learning mazes and other cognitive tests.[74] In subsequent tests, Dr. Dubal and her colleagues found people with the APOE-4 gene who had a higher than average amount of klotho did not exhibit extra clumps of plaques and tangles in the brain typically associated with Alzheimer's.[75] The researchers theorized klotho may slow the effects of carrying APOE-e4, perhaps by vitalizing the brains and making them biologically more youthful.[76] Given the impact of klotho on improving cognitive performance in mice some researchers are scrambling to develop safe therapeutic versions of injectable klotho for humans.

Furthermore, since altered levels of gamma-aminobutyric acid (GABA) have been observed in Alzheimer's, dementia and depression patients, some researchers are exploring potential drugs for impaired GABA receptors responsible for memory.[77] GABA is a complex inhibitory neurotransmitter that modulates cell-to-cell communication and facilitates chemical messaging within the brain.[78] A mood-regulating neurotransmitter used in about 20% of synapses in the nervous system, GABA helps fine-tune neural circuits in areas like the hippocampus, playing a key role in memory, motor control, and tackling anxiety.[79] GABA receptors foster homeostasis in the brain, with GABA-A receptors changing their configuration and composition when cells experience stress.[80] Meanwhile, other researchers are pushing the envelope, contemplating the prospects of using CRISPR for gene editing to prevent dementia.[81] For example, researchers are using

CRISPR to target GABA receptors with neurosteroids, chemicals, naturally occurring in the brain, that are involved in emotional and motivational brain networks.[82]

Rising cases of dementia and Alzheimer's Disease (AD) constitute a global health emergency, with all indicators pointing to a very grim future, especially for the aging population. Dementia is a primary cause of disability for persons over 65; it contributes about 11% of total years lived with disability for persons over 60 years old - more so than stroke, musculoskeletal disorders, heart disease, and all forms of cancer.[83] Accounting for about 60 – 80 percent of dementia cases, Alzheimer's disease (AD) currently afflicts 5.7 million Americans, and it is the sixth leading cause of death in the U.S., with the total rising a staggering 123% from 2000-2015.[84] Every 65 seconds, someone in the U.S. develops Alzheimer's, a number expected to double by 2050 when one American will develop the disease every 33 seconds.[85] The total number of cases of AD is expected to triple over the next thirty years, with the greatest increases projected to occur among Hispanic and African American populations.[86] The number of persons beyond age 65 who have Alzheimer's doubles every five years, and it is estimated that approximately one-third of all people over 85 may have Alzheimer's disease.[87] Currently, one in 10 people over 65 has Alzheimer's and 1 in 3 seniors currently is dying of it or related dementia.[88] It is also estimated that about 10-20% of older adults have mild cognitive impairment (MCI), the interim phase between the usual cognitive decline associated with normal aging versus the descent to dementia or Alzheimer's.[89] People with MCI are 2.5 times at risk of developing dementia.[90] There are gender and racial/ethnic disparities in the toll inflicted by Alzheimer's: women make up two-thirds of the cases, Hispanics (12%), and non-Hispanic whites (10 percent). [91] It is estimated that the disease affects Latinos in greater numbers relative to the general population, with a projected 600 percent spike by 2050.[92]

Economic costs are skyrocketing, casting a mushrooming pall on the nation's long-term financial security. The direct formal economic costs of dementia in the U.S. are estimated at $100 to $215 billion per year, mostly due to the high costs of institutionalization, with annual cost per patient averaging $42,000 to $56,000 annually.[93] Informal costs, including unpaid care by family members as well as caregivers' lost opportunity to earn income, are estimated at $18 billion.[94] Although the dementia crisis is expected to worsen very sharply in the coming years, society is grossly unprepared to confront the staggering magnitude of this looming challenge. In 2018, Alzheimer's care in the U.S. cost an estimated $277 billion, a figure expected to exceed a trillion dollars by 2050 - not including uncompensated care by over 16 million caregivers valued at over $232 billion.[95] Increasingly a global epidemic, about 50 million people are currently have dementia/Alzheimer's - projected to exceed 76 million by 2030 and approximately 135 million in 2050.[96] The current cost of care worldwide is estimated at $604 billion annually, a figure that excludes the efforts of caregivers.[97] Family caregivers, who typically work very long and lonely hours daily, experience high levels of psychological distress but are generally ignored and unsupported by policy makers. Only the 'lucky' few can find appropriate and affordable facilities to help them provide care for their loved ones. Thus, when Linda Grossman found Rosener House, a well-run adult day care facility to care for her husband with Alzheimer's, she called it a "godsend" and "a sanity saver" that lifted a "huge weight" from her shoulders.[98] She stated that finding supportive care for her husband allows her to have "a little bit of a life" because providing round the clock care is not just "emotionally exhausting," it could also be "physically taxing."[99] Barbara Kalt, the former director of Rosener House, thinks more needs to be done to support the millions of caregivers (many with full-time jobs) who are providing over a billion hours of uncompensated care.[100] The current and future challenges revolving around dementia prevention and have led some observers to call it "the greatest health challenge of our time."[101]

*****

Parkinson's Disease (PD) is a neurological disorder that progresses as dopamine-containing cells (the neurons of the pars compacta in the substantia nigra) are lost, effectively jeopardizing the brain's system for controlling movement and coordination.[102] While Parkinson's is a chronic condition, the disease typically progresses slowly, often beginning with relatively mild symptoms but steadily worsening over time to include severe motor impairments and other non-motor symptoms.[103] As the disease progresses, the availability of dopamine to the brain is sharply curtailed, and there is an increasing disengagement in proper signaling between the brain and the peripheral nervous system that controls muscles.[104] Over time, Parkinson's patients experience wide-ranging motor impediments including the following: extremely slow movement (bradykinesia); difficulties with posture, stability, balance, and coordination; freezing of gait; stiffness of the limbs and trunk; involuntary movements or dyskinesias (including tics, tremors, irregular and repetitive muscle movements); loss of physical movement (akinesia); dizziness while or after standing (orthostatic hypotension) and general postural instability - often resulting in falls and associated injuries.[105] In addition to asymmetrical motor fluctuations, patients may also contend with a range of non-motor symptoms, including urinary disturbances, bodily pain, loss of sense of smell or hyposmia, sleep disorders, rapid eye movements, tingling sensations in the extremities (paresthesia), constipation, and fatigue.[106] Communication difficulties include weakened speech muscles resulting in slurred speech (dysarthria), decreased volume of speech (hypophonia), stuttering (tachyphemia) as well as changes in tone, rhythm, rate and overall quality of speech.[107] Many PD patients suffer from swallowing disorders (deglutition and dysphagia), which increase the risk of aspiration pneumonia, considered the leading cause of death for persons who have Parkinson's.[108] The disease takes a cruel toll on mental health as patients may be plagued by neuropsychiatric disturbances, including wild mood swings, depression, hallucinations, delirium, and overt dementia, the latter particularly likely among older persons who have been ill for a protracted period.[109] Insufficient physical activity among many Parkinson's patients heightens the risk of osteoporosis and muscle weakness, resulting in a further deterioration of functional mobility that also exacerbates risk of falls and related injuries.[110] The progressive decline in motor and non-motor functioning, leads to a diminution of independence that drastically impacts the quality of life, often requiring extensive care. Parkinson's Disease affects about 500,000 to one million Americans, with 50,000 to 60,000 new cases diagnosed annually; worldwide, about seven to 10 million people are afflicted by the disease. [111]

Dr. David Irwin, a neurology professor at U Penn, maintains Parkinson's, like Alzheimer's, is a disease of "protein misfolding" because it is marked by minuscule clumps of unusually modified proteins in the CNS called Lewy bodies.[112] These aberrant aggregations in brain areas that control movement consist of alpha-synuclein proteins that have been transformed - cut, folded, and chemically altered – a process closely associated with neurodegeneration.[113] In addition to genetic predisposition in some cases, PD can be caused by brain inflammation, head trauma, stroke, and environmental factors such as pesticides, pollution, and toxins.[114] It is also thought that oxidative stress, marked by too many free radicals, can result in cellular and protein damage and contribute to Parkinson's and Alzheimer's disease.[115] Some have also expressed concern that deposits in the brain of the contrasting agent gadolinium, resulting from MRIs of breast tissue, may cause Parkinson's, dementia, and other neurodegenerative disorders.[116] As genome sequencing becomes more sophisticated, scientists are getting insights into genes that can cause rare inherited forms of PD or even trigger early onset, and the factors accelerate the death of brain cells.[117] There is also some overlap between Parkinson's disease dementia (PDD) and Lewy body dementia (LBD) as both share clinical and pathological parallels - the crucial difference being the timing of cognitive impairments vis-à-vis the one-year rule. [118] Parkinson's patients with motor problems for at least a year before the onset of cognitive impairment are diagnosed with PDD; in contrast, those who suffer mental impairments within a year of motor difficulties, or even before the start of motor problems are diagnosed with LBD.[119] Given its propensity to strike older people, Parkinson's is identified by the NIH as a major threat to brain health in the aging process:

the disease typically begins in the fifties or sixties, and there is increased incidence with advancing age.[120] A minority who develop the disease before 40 years are designated as having early-onset PD while those starting between 21 and 40 years are dubbed young-onset PD. [121] Persons afflicted before age 20 fall into the category of juvenile Parkinsonism, widely thought to have genetic origins.[122]

While there is no cure for Parkinson's, the centerpiece of clinical treatment is levodopa, a drug that nerve cells convert to dopamine; it temporarily ameliorates or reverses symptoms for a few years for some patients, but does not slow the underlying neurodegeneration.[123] Levodopa loses effectiveness as the disease progresses while also triggering severe side effects, including uncontrolled movements (dyskinesias) as well as on-off fluctuations in symptom control.[124] In some cases, physicians use Deep Brain Stimulation (DBS) – effectively, electrical excitation of brain cells in motor regions through implanted electrodes.[125] Other potential therapies include fetal tissue transplantation and the use of stem cells as well as induced pluripotent stem cells (iPSCs) from the patient's skin cells, to replace lost brain cells.[126] Possible therapeutic interventions may also involve the use of antioxidants (coenzyme Q10) and the fat molecule GM1 ganglioside to augment the capacity of nerve cells to produce neurotransmitters and enable molecular configurations for nerve cell survival.[127] Some researchers are also investigating the impact of PD on non-dopamine cells in the brain and their effect on non-motor symptoms – an area often overlooked in current treatment regimens.[128]

*****

II. The Dancing Brain: Hardwired to Move & Get into the Groove

Imagine for moment word leaked out some very brainy scientists were goosing up their multi-million-dollar facility with a fancy discotheque – for *research* purposes only! Think of all the snark and good-natured ribbing such breaking news would unleash. How many brain scientists does it take to get a party started? What's next? Neuroscientists curating musical selections, riffing, and mixing it up in the DJ's booth? Seriously? This is no laughing matter. Pioneering neuroscientists such as Dr. Helena Bronte-Stewart are charting new terrain and thinking imaginatively, not just outside the box, but discarding the old 'box' and building new structures from the ground up.[1] When Stanford University was planning a new neuroscience building, neuroscientist and former professional dancer, Dr.

Bronte-Stewart ensured the layout included a dance studio with a flexible floor and glass walls on two sides.[2] Together with another colleague, she obtained a grant to support a community dance program to improve brain health and tackle diseases like Parkinson's.[3]

Dance? We all know it. We have all seen it. We have all done "This thing, called [dance]...It swings ...It jives...It shakes all over like a jelly fish... ... gotta be cool, relax, get hip...And get on my track's ... Crazy little thing called [dance]." Imagine for a moment, the legendary Freddie Mercury grooving and crooning away. Across civilizations, dance has been a potent vehicle of creative expression, manifesting all aspects of the human condition, articulating through motion the fluid art of been, being, and becoming - the very stuff of consciousness itself. Perhaps Descartes should have stated: *I dance, therefore I am!* Etymologically linked to the Sanskrit "tan" as well as the French "danse," German "tanz," Italian "danza" or the Portuguese "danca," the dance - in any language - is at least as old as Homo Sapiens, and, certainly older than conventional speech.[4] Dubbed the universal language, dance is common to humans, animals, and birds, from little babes to mighty dinosaurs, cutting through cultural and other roadblocks, to create a shared domain of discourse. Dance capitalizes on spirited rhythmic movement to annotate the experience of being, interpreting, and broadcasting messages from the innards of the dancer, portraying the full panoply of human sensations in motion. Effectively the filmic chronicle of the mind, dance is an expression of the performer's inner matrix of feelings, thoughts, and appetites, making it an authentic and an aboriginal form of kinetic intercourse. Taking a mirror to the soul, dance reflects the participant's spirited engagement with consciousness, providing a creative outlet for externalizing the experience of the dancer's inner and external world. Like a spokesperson for the interior world, dance articulates, translates, and gives graphic voice and dramatic illustration of the deepest workings and musings of the mind – lending form and presence to consciousness. To paraphrase Rod Stewart, every movement tells a story.

The versatility of the dancer's body as a medium of art is also formed by the combined elements of force, flow, time, and space simultaneously.[5] In a transient feast of motion, the art of the dance is shaped by four principal elements: (1) flow - the amount of energy restricted within or released away from the center of the mover; (2) time - the speed of movement and manipulation of rhythmic patterns/measures; (3) space - floor patterns, direction, level and shape; and, (4) force – the effort, dynamics and weight resulting from energy outflow. [6] Through instantaneous emanations, dance moves communicate a dancer's message simultaneously and uniquely as the creator-artist and the work are bound together inextricably and indistinguishably. In what Suzanne Langer calls a "living and vital human experience," the dance casts the performer in constant dialogical engagement between the realms of thought and action, nature and nurture, being and becoming. [7] This kinetic dialectic is expressed as a continuous sequence of motion across time, in the course of "becoming the dance which it is, yet never fully the dance at any moment."[8] Embodied in an organic medium, all dance is movable and malleable, effectively a "plastic art" composed of "a spectacle of shifting patterns of created design" in a vivid interplay of flow, force, space and time.[9] Moreover, Jamake Highwater draws attention to the fluid spontaneity of dance, moving from organs of perception through kinesthetic sensing in our muscles, instantly linking sentience and movement. [10] In that sense, dance is the "spontaneous link between mentality, feeling, and movement," instantly and seamlessly combining thought and sentiment with nonverbal physical expression - a presentation of the mind in motion, fluidly integrating what was, is, and will be.[11]

Whether formal or informal, elegant or unrefined, the dance, the universal leveler – an art form equally accessible to the mighty and lowly, the urbane and the *sans culottes*. Expressions of dance range from the primitive and freewheeling exhibitions of rhythmic movements to more elaborate manifestations of dance as a more structured performance art. [12] A more formal approach to dance may emphasize the elegance, harmony, regularity, and precision in the "ordered movements of the body" or what Munro referred to as "an ordered sequence of moving visual patterns of line, solid shape, and color."[13] In its more regimented form, the dancer's body expresses itself in patterned applications and structured steps, delivering a highly choreographed performance to a rhythmic accompaniment. [14] Even in this technically rigid form, the prose and poetry of the body didactically combine message, rhetoric, speech, thought, and feeling with "dramatic intent, and aesthetic elements," to create moving spectacles.[15] For the causal dancer, the dance typically manifests itself in more freewheeling but equally communicative ways, expressing the sheer delight in the unrestrained "experiencing of movement" and "feeling the beat" for just plain fun and even play. [16] Even when perceived as unstructured, non-refined, and less articulate, all forms of the dance emanate from the rhythmic expression of inner feeling. [17]

*****

Until the last decade or so, scientists paid scant attention to the neurological impact of dance and often reacted with skepticism to claims about its therapeutic potential. More recently, there has been growing research interest in investigating the intricate mental coordination dancing entails and how dance can be integrated into comprehensive efforts to stem neurodegenerative decline.[18] As these efforts proceed apace, scientists are discovering the human brain is so attuned to rhythm that the brain itself is akin to a dance machine, the choreographer behind the curtain, the real star of the show.[19] No wonder neuroscientist and choreographer, Ivar Hagendoorn, unequivocally declared that while the limbs move, "it is the brain that dances." [20] Moreover, as researchers study the dancing brain, they are developing a clearer picture of how the elaborate neural architecture necessary for planning and executing complex dance moves is connected to sustaining brain health. Brain health is the capacity "to remember, learn, play, concentrate and maintain a clear, active mind; ... to draw on the strengths of your brain - information management, logic, judgment, perspective and wisdom," and to make the most of your brain and lessen the risks that come with aging.[21] Parenthetically, while the focus here is primarily brain health, movement, exercise, and dance, also affect the overall health of the body, including reducing the risks for conditions such as heart disease, cancer, and diabetes. For example, avoiding a sedentary lifestyle, and increasing physical activities reduces diabetes, bad LDL cholesterol, and high blood pressure, boosting the immune system and ensuring these dangerous conditions do not converge to harm the brain.[22] Similarly, if untreated, obesity and diabetes can disrupt the brain's insulin system and set in motion a series of reactions that increase the production and accumulations of plaques linked to brain damage associated with Alzheimer's and dementia.[23] Likewise, if untreated, depression can eventually fuel chronic inflammation, injure blood vessels, and obstruct blood flow in the brain, precipitating the decline of neural networks and sparking the onset of dementia or Alzheimer's.[24] It appears that a holistic approach that addresses the interplay of myriad health risks is key to ensuring brain health. Moreover, more researchers - even the really 'serious' types - now recognize that to prevail in the battle against neurodegenerative disorders such as dementia, Alzheimer's, and

Parkinson's, they must reckon with the intriguing relationship between dancing and the brain.

It is oft-stated that dancer-choreographer Martha Graham called dance "the plainspoken language of the brain."[25] She was mightily prescient. As we learn more about the brain's functioning, where complex dance-related tasks occur seamlessly across multiple spheres, we are discovering the treasure trove of wisdom in Graham's aphorism. The eons-long evolutionary processes that resulted in bigger and more complex brains have also produced an intricate neural architecture for imagining, planning and executing complicated dance moves.[26] Despite her uncontested claim as the first bi-pedal primate, it is a safe bet that Lucy was no Misty Copeland. About 3.2 million years ago, our most famous Australopithecus ancestor sported a brain that was slightly less than 500 cubic centimeters; for comparison, today's average adult human brain clocks in about 1400 cubic centimeters or 1.4 liters and weighs about three pounds.[27] Homo Erectus, who co-existed with early H. Sapiens until the cataclysmic Mt. Toba eruption 74,000 years ago, had a brain ranging from 600 -1100 cubic centimeters, enabling that distant kin to display more advanced human-like behaviors.[28] While H. Erectus used tools and developed more elaborate social groupings, his/her brain was rather inefficiently organized, and it did not allocate much space to regions that control language and speech.[29] Meanwhile, Homo Habilis achieved a modest expansion in brain size, including an enlargement of the Broca's area, the language-connected zone of the frontal lobe.[30] About 500,000 years ago, average brain size had reached 1000 cubic centimeters with a steady upward trajectory continuing for roughly another 300,000 years; by the age of H.

Sapiens, brains averaged about 1200 cubic centimeters (1.2 liters).[31] Today, our supercomputer of a dancing brain is a labyrinthine electro-chemical contraption of abstruse opacity, woven into a galactic network of a gazillion plus cells, and more. After several hit and miss calculations, we now have a reliable estimate of the number of brain neurons – 86 billion – thanks to neuroscientist Suzana Herculano-Houzel, who dissolved the brain into soup as part of her technique.[32] In addition, there may be up to 1000 trillion synaptic linkages between neurons and other cells, with an estimated 1000 to 10,000 synapses per typical neuron.[33] This circuitous network also contains tens of billions of glial cells supporting neurons and innumerable branches, receptors, and neurotransmitters for biochemical messaging.[34] Go figure.

In an article published in *Current Biology*, Kevin Laland and his colleagues suggest the dramatic expansion of the human neocortex that occurred about 200,000 years ago had a massive impact on our development as skillful and creative dancers imbued with a high degree of dance intelligence.[35] Marta Florio at Harvard University attributes the exponential growth of neurons in the neocortex (about 80% brain volume) to the gene, ARHGAP11b, which, when flicked on and intensely activated, leads to massive production of neurons.[36] This expansion of the neocortex also led to massive changes in brain regions required to adapt to complexity, perhaps helping H. Sapiens outwit our primate competitors – at least on the dance floor.[37] In that regard, the neocortex and the cerebellum play a pivotal role in motor functions related to dance, including exercising significant control over the motor neurons of the spinal cord and brain stem.[38] This epic development resulted in a brain more capable of planning complex thoughts and actions, including better problem solving, language learning, and enhanced communicative abilities.[39] In addition, humans became more adept at community-building by using social skills like dancing, having gained an edge in moving our hands and limbs purposefully, creatively, and communicatively.[40]

Dance uniquely illustrates the brain's ability to engage in parallel quantum processing across multiple regions instantaneously; the dancing brain seamlessly weaves "sensory information from multiple channels (auditory, vestibular, visual, somatosensory) and the fine-grained motor control of the whole body."[41] Kevin Laland and his colleagues theorize that as brains got bigger and better organized, the connections between various regions were enhanced - a critical development for our ability to dance with greater agility, creativity, and extraordinary spontaneity.[42] Axons in regions of larger brains have better access to target sites in other areas, thereby increasing their ability to influence different zones.[43] Using PET scans to analyze brain functioning, scientists find dance engages multiple brain regions simultaneously, including the following five areas that together make vital contributions to learning, mastering, recalling, and performing rhythmic movements with flow and force, in time, and across space.[44] (1) In the frontal lobe, the motor cortex helps the dancer analyze, plan, control, and execute every voluntary move spontaneously in immediate response to rhythmic tempo, structure, melodies, and patterns.[45] This is as true for a novice as it is for a virtuoso like an Alvin Ailey. (2) In the brain's parietal lobe, the somatosensory cortex oversees motor control and the proprioceptive system, facilitating hand-eye coordination, providing instant awareness of the body in space.[46] Think of Ginger Rodgers dancing backwards on heels yet conscious of her body in space and effortlessly finding Fred Astaire's hand without missing a beat! (3) Meanwhile, the basal ganglia collaborate with other regions to coordinate movement smoothly and ensure postural and balance control.[47] This enables you to pirouette like Misty Copeland or whirl like a dervish, without tumbling like bowling pins. (4) In the temporal lobe, the auditory cortex plays a vital role in processing sound - as we listen to music and connect it to stored memory in the hippocampus, while simultaneously processing cues from the primary visual cortex in the occipital lobe.[48] (5) The cerebellum incorporates inputs from the brain and spinal cord and helps to plan delicate and intricate motor actions with finesse and precision. [49] Visualize, for example, the mudras when dancing the Bharatanatyam. Thanks to the collaborative synchronization of these brain regions, we are quite adept at exhibiting 'dance intelligence,' including conceiving, learning, planning, recalling, and executing highly complex routines with versatility.[50] Our finely-tuned rhythmic brains, imbued with spontaneous links between the motor and auditory regions, integrating inputs from the forebrain, through the midbrain and the hindbrain, have enabled humans to emerge supreme in the evolutionary choreographic epic.[51]

In addition to its vast computational prowess, the brain also moonlights as a dance-music machine, with brain networks across multiple regions acutely attuned to, and fully engaged with sound and rhythm.[52] When sound waves strike the eardrum, they trigger additional vibrations of fluid waves in the cochlea. [53] This prompts about 15,000 hair cells or cilia to release neurotransmitters which stimulate the auditory nerve and send electrical signals to the auditory cortex. [54] Once it receives sound, the brain differentiates music from noise; without missing a beat, it seamlessly decodes and interprets such elements as pitch, chords, harmony, timbre, rhythmic structure and message. [55] As researchers Edward Large and Joel Snyder have shown, our brains are intensely rhythmic biological machines, whose patterns and neural oscillations seamlessly interact and synchronize with rhythms in the surrounding environment.[56] They contend that while listening to musical tones played at regular intervals, neural circuits reflect cyclic fluctuations in electrical field strength as brain networks analyze and react to rhythmic structures.[57] Large and Snyder surmised rhythmic communication takes place through spurts of high-frequency activity amongst various brain regions as neurons vibrate in reaction to rhythmic patterns. [58]

The unique interplay of dance and music in the brain probably arose from their fraternal and somewhat symbiotic origins as music and dance were most likely born together, perhaps out of some celebratory primordial rhythmic foot stomping or handclapping.[59] It is thought that the combination of dance and music reinforce each other in the brain, animating several regions across brain networks, including the reward centers that contribute to happy feelings throughout, courtesy of an infusion of dopamine.[60] Dopamine is a signaling molecule that carries signals between nerves in the brain, transmitting messages from neuron-to-neuron across tiny vacuums (synapses) onto receptors that signal the receiving neuron.[61] Dopamine neurons, produced in the substantia nigra and the ventral tegmental area of the midbrain, aka the brain's rewards center, are involved in pleasurable activities ranging from roller coasters and sex to dancing and alcohol.[62]

These neurons also play a key role in the brain's system for controlling movement and coordination, a matter of great consequence when it comes to unpacking the nature of neurodegenerative diseases like Parkinson's.[63] At a basic level, music enhances timing, coordination, synchronization, and entrainment to rhythm, helping dancers fine-tune their movements as they groove to the beat while adjusting instinctively to tempo and shifting patterns. But as neurologist John Krakauer of Columbia University wrote in the *Scientific American*, there is something even more extraordinary going when the brain synchronizes to music during the dance. Krakauer suggests the interplay of dance and music effectively creates a "pleasure double play" in the brain, igniting the mesolimbic pathway's reward zones and activating the cerebellum at the back, behind the brain stem.[64] By stoking reward centers from the orbitofrontal cortex to the ventral tegmental area (midbrain) and the ventral striatum in the forebrain, the dancing brain is awash with dopamine and other pleasure-giving biochemicals.[65] These feel-good neurotransmitters from dopaminergic pathways shape our moods and also affect brain health.[66]

Researchers have observed a dancer's brain lights up during dance, creating a rush very similar to the runner's high. Also, when listening to music that hits just the right notes, about two-thirds of people occasionally experience frissons, goosebumps, or aesthetic chills (dubbed skin orgasms) along their spine.[67] This phenomenon is more common in persons with more nerve fibers linking the auditory cortex to areas that process feelings (the anterior insular cortex) and shape reactions to rewarding experiences such as the ventral striatum's nucleus accumbens.[68]

Researchers also think when we observe others

dancing, we simultaneously experience an emotional and even joyful connection as similar brain areas are triggered when making or observing dance movements. [69] Innately synchronized to the performer's movements, the observer is, perforce, caught up in the brain's dance, as s/he follows the performer like a planet orbits the sun.[70] In this synchronized entanglement of performer and observer, the latter simulates the performance in the mind's eye; s/he anticipates and predicts moves with increasing pleasure, which could turn into a rush of euphoria when a dancer adroitly injects an unpredicted move that defies the internal imitation.[71] In an article published in *PLOS One*, Valarie Salimpoor and her colleagues at McGill uncovered an intriguing evolutionary connection between listening to music and dopamine release in the limbic system.[72] Using brain imaging, the researchers demonstrated that music, perceived as highly emotional, engaged the brain's reward system by triggering subcortical nuclei implicated in reward, motivation, and emotion. [73] For example, dopamine is released in the ventral striatum a few seconds before the "anticipation phase" or at "peak emotional moments" during performances when the listener experiences an aesthetic chill.[74] This finding appears to confirm Krakauer's view that reward is partially connected to anticipation or the correct "prediction of a desired outcome" – a desirable evolutionary trait for survival.[75] According to this approach, dopamine neurons effectively notated our accurate predictions and then rewarded us with the biochemical version of an attaboy or you-go-girl![76]

These feelings of joyfulness and emotional uplift associated with dancing are of great consequence for patients with neurological disorders. Since there are no cures for dementia, Alzheimer's, and Parkinson's, non-pharmacological interventions that provide relief and happiness from time to time could be the difference-maker. For example, the non-profit Creative Aging Mid-South has invested over $1 million for over 6,000 music and dance performances at senior centers for people with dementia to bring joy.[77] At one dance party at the Village in Germantown replete with greatest hits from yesteryear, Weezie, a 94-year-old woman with dementia, could be seen dancing on her wheelchair, rolling it forward to center stage, loving every minute of the show.[78] She was "grinning, clapping, and almost bouncing," singing "every verse" of the songs, "connecting to a time and place," that, but for the music, "might be lost to her forever."[79] As one Alzheimer's patient danced away in a seemingly carefree manner during one of the programs, he told Meryl Klein, the program's director, "I may die tomorrow, but I'll die happy."[80] After witnessing the transformations wrought by music and dance at the facility, Brenda Olloway, activities director at The Village at Germantown, stated: "It's a better pill than any medicine." [81]

Besides dopamine, movement, dance, and other forms of exercise trigger a spike in serotonin, noradrenaline, GABA, and glutamate, neurotransmitters that regulate signaling and transmit biochemical messages throughout the brain.[82] Meanwhile, serotonin, with its intricate signaling system with over 15 distinct receptors (attached proteins), also acts as a neurotransmitter. [83] Serotonin prompts brain cells to fire messages that, among other things, boost the capacity to cope with stress, adversity, and helping us to avoid or manage the pitfalls of depression.[84] Physical activities, including dancing, can also activate brain pathways that result in increased production of gamma-aminobutyric acid (GABA), a complex inhibitory mood-regulating neurotransmitter.[85] As noted earlier, GABA is used in about 20% of synapses in the nervous system and facilitates chemical messaging within the brain, fine-tuning neural circuits in areas like the hippocampus, playing a key role in memory, motor control, and tackling anxiety.[86] GABA receptors foster homeostasis in the brain, with GABA-A receptors changing their configuration and composition when cells experience stress.[87] A study by UC Davis researchers demonstrated, physical activity activates the metabolic pathways that replenish deficiencies in neurotransmitters such as GABA and glutamate.[88] The researchers used nuclear magnetic resonance spectra to image the brains of 38 exercisers who had reached about 85% of their predicted maximum heart rates while cycling on stationary bikes.[89] They found that while GABA and glutamate levels remained unchanged among non-exercisers, levels increased among exercisers, particularly in the visual cortex and the anterior cingulate cortex, helping regulate heart rate, emotion, and some cognitive functions.[90] The researchers theorized the brain uses some of the extra energy obtained from glucose and other carbohydrates during exercise to make more neurotransmitters.[91] Researchers think GABA plays a key role in diminishing the activity of neurons in both the brain and CNS as well as significant involvement in gut health. [92] For example, Elizabeth Gould and her colleagues at Princeton University found that unlike sedentary mice, brains of running mice released GABA in response to stress.[93] This GABA release tamped down neural excitement by reining in excitable neurons, effectively reorganizing the brain to be more adaptive and resilient to stressors.[94] In effect, GABA downshifts the brain, resulting in greater calm, lower stress, relaxation, reduced pain, better sleep, and more balanced moods.[95] Since altered GABA levels have been observed in various mood disorders, dementia, and Alzheimer's, some researchers are targeting new drugs on impaired GABA receptors.[96] Dopamine, serotonin, GABA, and other neurotransmitters effectively act together as natural mood regulators - akin to synthetic antidepressants and other similar prescription drugs for mood disorders such as depression and anxiety. [97]

Scientists also think exercising initiates the production of brain-derived neurotrophic factor (B.D.N.F.) - dubbed the "Miracle-Gro for your brain" by neuro-psychiatrist John Ratey at Harvard medical.[98] BDNF fuels the production of new neurons in the hippocampus contributing to a rich environment where neurons thrive and forge new interconnections between cells, resulting in greater synaptic density. [99] In experiments with lab animals, researchers have shown how exercise prompts production of the protein B.D.N.F., which supports brain metabolism, helping new cells grow and promoting the development and vitality of hippocampal neurons.[100] Furthermore, researchers at the University of British Columbia found the volume of brain regions that control thinking and memory (the prefrontal cortex and medial temporal cortex) is more extensive in exercisers versus non-exercisers.[101] Even moderately intense physical activity, with aerobic components that get the heart and sweat glands pumping, can prompt the brain to produce BDNF and other growth factors contributing to an enlargement of cognitive regions by accelerating adult hippocampal neurogenesis.[102] This activation of brain metabolism effectively promotes the growth of new blood vessels in the brain, and enhances the health, abundance, and resilience of new brain cells.[103] Some researchers think practitioners of more vigorous High-Intensity Interval Training (HIIT) workouts that incorporate brief and extremely robust bursts of physical activity are more likely to increase BDNF levels substantially.[104] It is thought that HIIT workouts are more likely to cause the pituitary gland to release human growth hormone, thereby improving neurotransmitter levels and production of much higher levels of BDNF and noradrenaline. [105] Nonetheless, the general view is that even moderate but consistent physical activity impacts the brain's neuroplasticity, boosts the size of the hippocampus, enhances memory recall, and supports the homeostasis of the central and peripheral nervous systems.[106] In plain terms, your brain will be a tad bigger, more nimble, and a smidgen smarter, and you just might purchase an extra measure of protection against the ravages of Father Time, to boot.

Recall from earlier that researchers looking into drugs for Alzheimer's and dementia are taking a serious look at the super-powerful hormone klotho. [107] However, even without the clinical version, moderate and regular exercise, including dancing, can help you increase Klotho production, a key ingredient in your arsenal to stave off neurodegenerative decline. In an article published in *Experimental and Therapeutic Medicine,* Naichun Ji and colleagues at the Xi'an Medical University found exercise could delay aging and extend healthy longevity by increasing the Klotho gene expression in mice brain and kidney tissues.[108] The researchers theorized klotho helps avoid the damage to the brain and kidneys caused by harmful Reactive Oxygen Species (ROS), thereby enhancing brain metabolism and supporting healthy longevity.[109] Furthermore, in an article published in *AJP Heart and Circulatory Physiology,* Tomoko Matsubara and his colleagues also found aerobic exercise training increased plasma Klotho concentrations and reduced arterial stiffness among participants.[110] Meanwhile, writing in *Frontiers in Physiology,* Keith Avin and his colleagues at the University of Pittsburgh have suggested Klotho expression may be modulated by skeletal muscle activity, noting levels are upregulated in reaction to vigorous exercise.[111] Avin and other researchers observe these findings all have significant implications for understanding the anti-aging effects of exercise.[112] Although some scientists are exploring the possibilities of klotho-based therapeutic interventions, we need not wait; we can elevate klotho levels, stave off neural decay, and extend healthy longevity through movement, exercise, and dance.[113]

The hormone irisin is also receiving greater attention as a significant factor in understanding how exercise improves brain health and reduces the risk of neurodegenerative disorders.[114] Named after the god's messenger in Greek mythology, Irisin is produced by muscles during exercise, and it triggers biochemical reactions (mostly involving energy metabolism) throughout the body. [115] More recently, researchers have found irisin in the brain, including evidence it was produced inside the brain. [116] While researchers have found high levels of irisin in brains of people who died free of dementia, it is barely noticeable in people who had died with dementia or Alzheimer's. [117] When researchers investigating the impact of irisin on neurodegenerative disorders infused a heavy dose of the hormone in mice with dementia, it improved memory test performance.[118] Next, researchers blocked irisin production in healthy mice and then gave them dementia; without irisin in their brains, the once-healthy mice suffered a rapid neurodegenerative decline.[119] When healthy mice exercised, irisin levels in the brain were boosted; when brains of exercisers were exposed to beta-amyloid, they were more resilient and performed better on memory tests than the sedentary control group.[120] However, when researchers blocked irisin production in mice and exposed them to beta-amyloid, they did not exhibit the cognitive benefits of exercise.[121] Since Alzheimer's involves changes in how brain cells use energy, researchers think exercise may have a protective effect by heightening irisin levels and alleviating or even forestalling the disease.[122]

Another way that movement, exercise, and dance make the brain more youthful and responsive is contributing to the thickness of white matter health and slowing myelin shrinkage.[123] White matter, comprising about

60% of the brain, consists of myelinated nerve fibers grouped into tracts carrying nerve signals between brain cells; axons or filaments represent connections between brain processing centers creating an elaborate communications network.[124] Meanwhile, constituting about 40% of the brain, gray (pinkish) matter is comprised of cell bodies, dendrites, and axon terminals of neurons; it is the locus of all synapses and represents information processing centers in the brain.[125] The growth and thickness of white matter are critical for maintaining the brain's processing speed and its ability to absorb, analyze, and react to new information. [126] Denser white matter, especially in the all-important fornix, contributes to much more rapid and efficient information processing and transmission of messages between neurons.[127] Processing speed slows with aging, perhaps due to the fraying of the brain's white matter and attendant myelin shrinkage.[128] As myelin shrinks, it leads to less dense white matter; sparser and less effective white matter cells result in a slower transmission of messages between neurons in one region to another.[129] This problem contributes to the memory deficits afflicting up to one-third of older people, including a decline in declarative memory (retrieving stored facts, events, etc.) and challenges in learning new things, multitasking, recalling names and numbers.[130] Demyelination can signify microvascular or small ischemic blood vessel disease; coupled with the white matter damage, it is associated with dementia and poor motor functioning among the elderly.[131] Exercise can enhance myelin sheath regeneration: for example, in one study of the brains of 74 people with MS, researchers showed had a significant therapeutic impact, effectuating substantial changes in brain tissue.[132] When researchers examined the participants after exercise, they found noticeable differences in nineteen participants' brains, including significant

cortical thickening that indicated preservation or

regeneration of brain tissue.[133] Similarly, Isobel

Scarisbrick at Mayo Clinic found exercise also helped

reverse the harmful impacts of a high fat and sugar diet

on the health of myelinating cells.[134] Meanwhile,

another article published in the *Journal Nature*

Neuroscience shows myelin levels are elevated in the

course of complex brain processes and activities,

especially those that involve memorization and

replication as well as the execution of complex

movement sequences involving dozens of muscles.[135]

Some healthy seniors are already ahead of the experts,

'medicating' themselves with the novelty, energy, and

therapeutic potency of dance. Consider, for example,

two participants at a line dance workout program for

seniors throughout the Dallas area conducted by

instructor Cyndi Dorber.[136]   First, a woman named Louise, who took up line dancing class for the first time, at age eighty-five, made a tremendous amount of progress within a year, especially given that as she put it, "I couldn't dance a step. I was raised a Baptist. Dancing wasn't allowed."[137]   A year later, she was confident enough to offer some lessons: "Your brain and your feet have to work together...You have to listen to the beat and pay attention to the steps. It helps you mentally as well as physically... And if you miss a step, it's no big deal. You just look at the person next to you and catch up. The important thing is that you're moving for an hour." [138] Meanwhile, Peggy Smith, a seventy-three-year-old dancer at the same workshop, shared these words of wisdom: "...Life can begin in your 70s. But you have to work at it. There are always new things to learn, new places to go, new things to try, new people to meet. Everyday can be a new adventure. You just have to have the right attitude."[139] Louise and Peggy

Smith are trendsetters, and we should all be inspired by

their avid interest in the mental and physical benefits of

dancing. The sedentary older adult is more susceptible

to demyelination. Inactivity heightens the risk of

developing plaques in brain white matter, signaling

potentially destructive white matter disease (white

matter hyperintensities), with lesions that appear as

bright spots on MRI images.[140] In this context, learning

and memorizing intricate dance sequences (like Ms.

Peggy Smith and Louise are modeling above) may help

improve the health of white matter and ward off

demyelination. Given the association between dementia

and myelin shrinkage, there may be opportunities to

delay or slow the progression of dementia with the help

of dancing and other exercises.[141]

Why do dervishes not tumble over when they spin in what seems like forever? Merry-go-rounds leave many of us dizzy, even after the spinning stops, because of the signals sent to the cerebellum by the vestibular organs, the fluid-filled chambers of the inner ear. [142] That sense of dizziness persists as the vestibular fluid continues to move and send signals that make it appear as if we are still in motion. [143] If dizziness is inevitable, why are certain people able to spin for hours on end without tumbling over like bowling balls? As Yuliya Nigmatullina and her colleagues at Oxford University found, regular practice as occurs in ballet training (or whirling like a dervish) can initiate significant changes in the cerebral cortex that render dancers less susceptible to dizziness or even falling.[144] In an article published in *Cerebral Cortex*, the researchers showed that as dancers become more proficient at pirouetting, their sustained conditioning changes their vestibular reactions, giving them an extraordinary ability to pay less attention to inputs from their vestibular organs.[145] Frequent and sustained pirouetting effectively changes vestibular processing in the brain, enabling the dancer to spin like a dervish with little or no feeling of vertigo.[146] These dancers can suppress vertigo because of a significant reduction in vestibular signaling and differential sensory processing of the vestibular perception and the reflexive vestibular-ocular-reflex (VOR).[147] The transformation is perceptible: when the brains of ballet dancers are scanned, MRIs show the signal processing area in the cerebellum is significantly smaller relative to the general population.[148] To the extent that dance training reduces dizziness and improves balance, the dance could help older adults avoid life-threatening falls and related injuries.

*****

Are we evolutionarily hardwired to dance? It is often said that dance is as old as Homo Sapiens, but it is unclear when and why Homo Sapiens did the first jig. Unlike other art forms, the dance's intrinsic transience and the absence of physical evidence make it more difficult to reconstruct an evolutionary timeline. In some ways, this ephemeral aspect of dance is captured by fleeting floor paintings (mandalas) fashioned by India's outcaste Pullavas. Mandalas comprised of eight cobra-hooded snakes were created during ritual dance ceremonies to help high caste families propitiate their serpent deities and ward off ill-fortune; they were promptly destroyed after the ceremony, leaving no trace.[149] Nonetheless, anthropologists always say that dancing is as old as man, giving dance a starting point that goes back at least 300,000 years. In 2017 Jean-Jacques Dublin and his colleagues at the Max Planck

Institute for Evolutionary Anthropology identified what they believed to be the earliest known ancestor of modern humans, thought to be about three hundred and fifty thousand years old at Jebel Irhoud in Morocco.[150] While it is not known when humans first dance, there is evidence of dancing and related creative activity going back at least 100,000 years and other significant finds in the Upper Paleolithic era. [151] In India's Bhimbetka caves inhabited as far back as 100,000 years ago, archaeologists have identified some of the earliest rock art paintings of communal dancers and animals. First discovered by archaeologist V.S. Wanakar in 1975, Bhimbetka Rock Shelters, located in India's Madhya Pradesh region (home of the Bhopal Union Carbide chemical catastrophe), are now considered a prominent UNESCO World Heritage site.[152] Before this significant find, the most significant physical proof of ancient ritual dance art from an earlier period was a Paleolithic dwelling found in France in 1940 at Le Mas D'Azil in southern France.[153] The incredible trove of cave art consists of rock paintings depicting masked dancers, war dances, dancing shamans, hunters, and various animals thought to be as old as 35,000 years.[154] Similarly, at the caves of Chauvet and Lascaux as well as in caves near Palermo Sicily, archaeologists have identified Paleolithic-era ritual depictions of animals.[155] Other recent archaeological excavations in Africa and Asia have also opened promising new vistas of research for scholars looking for the physical evidence of ritual dance and to gain a better understanding of our humanistic heritage. For example, the discoveries of 164,000-year old pigment ocher and shells, and a painting workshop at the 100,000-year old Blombos Cave, both in South Africa, provided new insights into our evolutionary lineage.[156] The decorative items thought to be finery or jewelry introduced the possibility that artistic and creative expressions, including ritual dance, occurred in Africa as far back as that early period.[157] Likewise, at Botswana's Rhino Cave, researchers discovered a rock panel estimated at 65,000-70,000 years-old that suggests ritual dance practices invoking spiritual forces. [158] Meanwhile, researchers in the Indonesian island of Sulawesi found seven limestone caves in 2016, containing paintings of hands and figurative animal depictions estimated to be 39,900 years old.[159] As Jean Clottes, a world-renowned cave expert, observed, these findings suggest symbolic thinking and creative expression have been a widespread and deeply established part of our humanistic heritage.[160] Not to be outdone, it also appears that our Neanderthal 'cousins' were also engaged in singing and dancing and left their own evidence of symbolic ritual art, to boot. [161] Researchers now maintain European Neanderthals possessed much higher cognitive and creative abilities than previously thought. They point to evidence that Neanderthals probably performed complex tasks, including herding animals for prey and using pitch processed from tree bark in an environment without oxygen.[162] In 2018, archaeologists discovered the La Pasiega, Maltravieso, and Ardales caves in Spain, which contain what are thought to be the world's oldest cave paintings by Neanderthals. [163] In an article published in the journal *Science* in 2018, the researchers noted the presence of Neanderthal art, including ornamented seashells (dated to about 115,000 years ago) and hand stencils of ritual figures including animals (created about 66,000 years ago) - significant evidence of symbolic thinking, creative expression and artistic sensibility.[164] With some evidence of cross-breeding between Neanderthals and H. Sapiens, the evolutionary ladder of dance may have some unusual twists and shouts, including a possible exchange of dance moves between Neanderthals and our kind.[165]

The cumulative evidence from ongoing research tends to confirm Darwin's assessment in the *Descent of Man*, about rhythm being a universal trait shared by all animals.[166] It appears this was true, even dinosaurs! According to a study published in *Scientific Reports*, physical evidence suggests dances of courtship and mating may have occurred among the ancient ancestors of birds, dinosaurs, millions of years ago![167] Researchers found giant gouges or scrapes (double-furrow markings and multiple tracks resembling those of Atlantic puffins or ostriches) at three sites in Dakota Sandstone of Colorado.[168] The find and subsequent analysis suggest that non-avian theropods or dinosaurs participated in courtship-like mating ritual dance observed in today's bird-of-paradise, including creating fancy leks or lairs to flaunt their wares.[169] Before the ubiquity of dancing animals on YouTube, one had to depend on accounts of scientists and anthropologists who often spent very long hours waiting to capture the moment for their reports. In a lab study in Tenerife of chimps, psychologist Wolfgang Kohler saw a female chimp dance excitedly as she hopped first on one leg, then on the other, then whirled rapidly with arms horizontally stretched out, mimicking a dance of the locals. [170] Later, he witnessed a bona fide round dance by the chimps, who formed a circle around a post, moving in an orderly manner, walking then trotting, then stomping with one foot.[171] Some donned ornaments (strings, vines, and the like) while stamping their feet to make music akin to a gorilla's boisterous and rhythmic chest-thumping. In another account, it was reported a cock performed dance-like moves, hopping about with wings extended and spreading out of tails, even synchronizing its movement with other chickens.[172] A report from Australia described a quadrille-like dance by hundreds of stork-like birds as they advanced and retreated, raising their legs high up and standing on their toes and occasionally bowing.[173] The creatures formed an encirclement, cavorting elegantly, heads bobbing in time, then forming a "great prancing mass," their necks pushed up and backs swaying, suddenly moving apart and then beginning anew.[174]

From dancing dinosaurs to dancing chimps, it appears we are all hardwired to dance. Like Darwin, Peter Cook of Emory University contends rhythm is virtually universal, part and parcel of a long evolutionary lineage. [175] Cook maintains rhythm is fundamental to life and hardwired, going back to the evolution of the brain itself; he argued entraining to rhythm was likely rooted in an ancient well-heeled mechanism intricately connected to how brains communicate. [176] In that regard, he maintained the "neural mechanisms underpinning flexible beat keeping" are much more broadly distributed throughout the animal kingdom than previously believed.[177] Moreover, Cook also argued following an auditory beat is not the only form of rhythm despite this being the focus of anthropocentric research. [178] A wide array of examples illustrate the prevalence of rhythm in the natural world, including: "the synchronous flash of the lustful firefly; or the lockstep of cheetah and gazelle; the ease with which millions of bats move together like living smoke in the night sky; the highly coordinated hunts of wolves and orcas; and the intricate mating dances of tropical birds."[179] As Cook posits, all members of the animal kingdom, as part of a shared evolutionary heritage, possess and exhibit innate abilities and propensities to both "sense rhythm and use it socially." [180] They do so according to their particular contextual need and not necessarily in activities that resemble dancing (as we know it), such as co-foraging activities or exotic mating rituals. [181] Cook maintains these rhythmic abilities certainly be found in close relatives like monkeys or apes.[182] However, other beneficiaries include even distant family tree kin like ring-legged fiddler crabs (waving claws in dance-like group displays) and foot-flagging frogs that signal rhythmically with their feet. [183] While some suggest certain animals seem really poor at detecting rhythmic patterns and even appear to lack "sensitivity to rhythms" (e.g., zebra finches), Cook argues that could simply be because researchers have not yet developed the right tests to assess rhythmic sensibilities of certain animals, particularly if they do not sense or feel rhythm like humans do. [184] Detecting rhythm among some species could require extra motivation, better assessment techniques, and perhaps a different way of looking at the question, including a broader perspective and maybe less ethnocentrism.[185] Setting aside the fracas about entraining to rhythm resolved by Patel Aniruddh's groundbreaking research on Snowball, the dancing cockatoo, we find plentiful evidence of dance in the animal world.[186]

As a BBC feature titled Ten Dazzling Dancers of the Natural world vividly illustrated, humans do not hold a monopoly of rhythm. [187] For example, Madagascar's Verreaux's sifaka (a lemur) has a dazzling dance-walk move after it occasionally descends from its treetop homes, cavorting gracefully in a sideways ballet-like step, arms held out for balance. [188] Incidentally, due to its very upright posture, disproportionately long legs, and short arms, walking on fours is not quite feasible. [189] Alternatively, consider the shrew mum's protective

dance as she steers her enormous litter in a septuplet
conga line; each youngster bites the top of the tail of the
shrew in front, ensuring all baby shrews safe and
sound.[190] Elsewhere, the large blood red sea slug of the
Indo-Pacific Ocean and the Red Sea ripples the delicate
edges of its mantle when swimming, thrusting its body
back and forth it propels itself upwards. [191] The process
evokes a flamenco dancer's swishing skirt, hence the
name 'The Spanish Dancer.'[192] Incidentally, while most
humans necessarily link music and dance, including
"mentally" dancing while listening to music, some
dancing birds (e.g., species of bird-of-paradise)"
perform dance displays without singing.[193] Meanwhile,
others such as lyrebirds (Menura novaehollandiae) will
sing without dancing and dance without singing.[194]

Dancing babies? Darwin's observation in the Descent of
Man that we have an innate propensity to enjoy music

and dance has been validated by studies that show even newborns and fetuses in the womb move to music. [195] Contemporary research on dance is showing that we are all rhythmic creatures, hardwired to respond to music, to dance, even before we could utter a word. Until recently, the conventional view was that little tots were incapable of synchronizing to a beat before they reached three years old. [196] Even in rare instances where children younger than four showed dancing ability, it was thought they were limited in their ability to experience music and could typically only move "at one tempo close to their preferred tempi."[197] Yet, in recent years, researchers began paying more attention to the evidence that babies may be hardwired to dance from early on and that they may be quite capable of learning dance moves and improvising at much younger ages than previously thought. [198] Over the past twenty years or so, significant new research has contributed to our understanding of how infants' brains synchronize to music, opening new horizons in our understanding of the origin and import of dance in the course of human evolution and development. [199] For example, researchers studying the development of human brains discovered that six-month-old babies are more proficient than adults at recognizing complex musical rhythms. It is also thought that by the time babies turn one, their ears are attuned to the sounds and rhythms of their culture.[200] The studies conducted by Sandra Trehub, a psychologist at the University of Toronto at Mississauga, and her colleagues also show that in addition to being more familiar with the music of their heritage, infants are more adept than adults at discerning the intricate patterns and rhythms of foreign music.[201] For example, one-year-old babies who listened to Balkan tunes several times a day over a period of weeks were more successful at identifying errors on those rhythms compared to adults who received similar exposure. [202] Based on this research, Trehub and her colleagues suggest that by engaging in interactive learning such as integrating dance classes and the study of complex foreign rhythms, adults can likewise enhance their skills, refining the ability to discern errors such as a missing beat.[203]

Meanwhile, Marcel Zentner and Tuomas Eerola of the University of York in England conducted an extensive review of rhythmic engagement in infancy in a groundbreaking study involving 120 infants between 5 months and two years old.[204] In research published in the *Proceedings of the National Academy of Sciences,* the researchers concluded that babies respond to rhythm/beat and tempo (not just the melody), suggesting babies may have an innate predisposition to dance.[205] The study also showed that babies who were sitting on a parent's lap responded with more rhythmic

movements or dancing when exposed to music

(recordings of classical music, rhythmic drumbeats)

than they reacted to speech. [206] Additionally, another

groundbreaking study conducted by Fuji Watanabe and

his colleagues in Japan of three four-month-olds

exposed to (of all things) music by the Backstreet Boys

showed babies clearly and simultaneously

demonstrated limb movements and vocalizations.[207] In

addition, two of the babies demonstrated they could

synchronize to the musical beat as they engaged in

remarkable increases in the rhythmic moves through

kicking or arm-waving consistent with the tempo of the

music. [208] Furthermore, research published by Adena

Schachner and her colleagues demonstrates that older

babies (8-12 months) but not younger ones (5-8

months) have the capacity to discern bad dancing as in

when the visual track was mismatched (asynchronous)

with the audio track, effectively discriminating matching stimuli from mismatching stimuli.[209] By demonstrating that 8-12-month-old infants perceive musical and audiovisual synchrony, the researchers provided illuminative insights on dance as a natural and shared heritage of even the littlest humans.[210]

In addition, using sophisticated new technologies, researchers have been able to reach further back in time, even to pre-natal babies in the womb, to understand why humans have a disposition to rhythm and dance.[211] Today, researchers can see "overt signs" that babies are trying to "engage in the music by singing along, clapping, and moving their bodies." [212] The researchers used an MRI scan with algorithms, magnetic fields, and radio waves to create ultra-high-resolution images of the fetus. [213] It showed a fetus as young as 20-weeks old was dancing, moving around, stretching its arms, turning its head from side to side, and kicking the mother's belly. [214] According to Dr. Laurel Trainor, babies' auditory systems function from the sixth prenatal month, and so they can hear the world around them and even form musical memories while still inside the womb.[215] Meanwhile, Istvan Winkler and Henkjan Honing, researchers at the Institute for Psychology of the Hungarian Academy of Sciences and Music, contend newborn infants can detect the regular beat in music.[216] Their research claims beat induction, "fundamental to the origins of music," is either innate or learned in the womb. Other researchers have found babies can hear and remember music even while in the womb; they can also recall the tempo and timbre of music previously heard.[217] Babies also choose "consonance over dissonance" and are more likely to prefer the female voice - especially in the high-energy singsong tone of motherese.[218] As Indian dance therapist Tripura Kashyap states, dance is innate such that even without lessons, observation, or imitation, "you start dancing even before you are born, in your mother's womb when you kick or move."[219] Whereas our disinclination to exercise may have evolutionary origins, as Harvard's Daniel Lieberman has suggested, dancing is the total opposite.[220] Obtaining the benefits of exercise through dance is fun and pleasant; it is also natural from an evolutionary perspective because humans, even newbies, are hardwired to dance and enjoy music.[221]

*****

Some researchers have also found some evidence of dance propensities in our genes. In an article published in the *American Journal, Public Library of Science Genetics*, Richard Ebstein and his colleagues found evidence indicating dancers are endowed with genes that contribute to greater social expression and heightened spirituality. [222] The researchers at the Hebrew University of Jerusalem maintain dancers show consistent differences in variants of two genes involved in the transmission of information between nerve cells related to dancing. [223] The first gene, the serotonin transporter, regulates serotonin levels and is vital to spiritual experience and correlates with altered states of consciousness; the second, the vasopressin receptor 1a, modulates social communication and bonding. [224] The researchers concluded 'dancer types' demonstrated greater communicativeness of a "symbolic and ceremonial" nature and stronger spirituality.[225] Recent technological advances have also enabled scientists to retrieve ancient human DNA from a fossil dating back 400,000 years.[226] Perhaps somewhere in the amber-filled labyrinth of fossilized DNA, there lies a genetic clue that further clarifies some of the puzzling questions about dance.

Researchers speculate music and dance were most likely born together, perhaps out of some joyous primordial rhythmic foot stomping or handclapping and diverse 'rhythms' such as chest-thumping, tongue-clicking, chanting, rapping, guttural sounds, or even the thrashing of twigs.[227] In an article published in *Current Biology,* Kevin Laland and his colleagues hypothesized that dance might have originally served as "an ethnic marker that promoted within-group identity and alliances."[228] As dance evolved, researchers theorize it also took on more community-building functions, including communicating religious and historical knowledge and facilitating sexual display for mate selection and procreation. [229] For example, researchers at Oxford University who investigated the connection between dance and social bonding noted that because dance is "intrinsically cooperative in nature," it played a central role in the development of human communities. [230] The researchers theorized that dance fostered community-building by serving "the evolutionary function of encouraging social bonds, cooperation and prosocial behaviours between group members."[231] As Steven Mithen, author of "The Singing Neanderthals," contends, the innate instinct to enjoy music, sing and dance helped foster healthy social bonds and was gradually encoded into our genome over time.[232]

*****

The hardwiring, and the yearning, for dance and perhaps even party the night away, do not stop just because one has Alzheimer's or dementia. In a classic Gotham-style initiative that grabbed worldwide attention, the Hebrew Home for the Aged at Riverdale,

New York, operated a unique and "revolutionary" late night dance party for senior citizens with dementia.[233] One of the beneficiaries of this groundbreaking approach was Maria Navarro, an 85-year-old grandmother with dementia who loved the salsa dancing leading to headlines such as "Dementia Patients Party Through the Night."[234] After all else had seemed to fail, her son Paul Navarro enrolled his mother in the program, which quickly became her home-away-from-home. For Ms. Navarro, participation in the program was "life-altering," helping her cope with insomnia, fear, and loneliness, and, above all, she no longer had to wake up her son every night for "the smallest of items." [235] With a full range of activities from 7 pm to 7 am, including music, dancing, art class, midnight strolls, massages, field trips to restaurants and theaters, one participant told Good Morning America, "... here we are a family."[236] As the program director Deborah Messina shared, "Our philosophy is that we're engaging their behavior and we're letting it happen. So, if someone wants to, you know, get up and walk and pace at 3 o'clock in the morning, we're going to engage that behavior because their internal clocks are so different." [237] Shortly after she joined, Paul observed a noticeable transformation in her mother. She literally became "a different person and noticeably more alert" and made new friends, bonding with a group of Spanish-speaking women who enjoyed gossip and each other's company. [238] As Mr. Navarro stated, "...my mother's happy and I couldn't be happier...Sometimes, I wonder who has the more active social life, my mother or me." [239] Such accounts of significant transformations of dementia and Alzheimer's patients arising from dance and musical interventions continue to pique researchers' interest.

III. Studies 'Show,' Dancers Experience

When the University of Washington Brain and Wellness Center (UW-MBWC) asked several people about their favorite "hobby" to enhance or sustain brain health, several notable answers centered on dance.[1] Elisabeth Lindley, a registered nurse practitioner at UW-MBWC wrote about her passion for learning ballroom dancing, having taken tango lessons with her husband while also looking forward to trying the waltz.[2] She attested to the mental benefits of dance, noting, "There's just so many things to keep track of: the music, where to step next, where my partner is, trying not to run into the other dancers. It's been a fun way to meet new people, get some exercise, and keep challenging my brain."[3] Tap dancing hits the spot for Erin Bowls, a Research Associate at Kaiser Permanente Washington Health

Research Institute, who wrote: "I love tap dancing. I drop in to classes at my local dance studio, where I am constantly challenged to pick up new steps and remember old ones. It's great exercise and extra fun with a great group of ladies."[4] Meanwhile, Marigrace Becker, Program Manager, Community Education and Impact at UW MBWC lauded the brain health benefits of contra dancing, writing: "My favorite brain healthy hobby is contra dancing! I always come away with a huge smile on my face from meeting friendly people, it's a great workout, plus takes a lot of concentration to quickly learn the moves of each dance."[5] Dr. Kristoffer Rhoads, a neuro-psychologist at the MWBC, maintained the learned sequences of movement in square dancing helped activate long-term memory, stating, "the complex cross-body movements of dancing recruit the procedural memory system and give it a work out."[6] Dr. Rhoads suggested engaging the procedural memory system through complex dances is beneficial because "It's also the form of memory that stays intact longer in people with Alzheimer's disease… and it may help people compensate for losses in short-term memory.[7]

The lived experiences of passionate dancers illuminate and vivify studies that show the potent impact of dance on the brain. In an article in the *New England Journal of Medicine* (2003), researchers examined how cognitive and physical activities impacted the risk of dementia among 469 persons over 75 who were dementia-free at the base line.[8] The participants engaged in cognitive activities like reading, playing board games and musical instruments as well as physical activities such as golf, swimming, bicycling, bowling, walking, and housework. [9] After the 21-year study period, the researchers found a significant association between a higher level of participation in leisure activities and cognitive activities and a reduced risk of Alzheimer's disease and vascular dementia, even after adjusting for baseline cognitive status.[10] Yet, among the physical activities included in the study, dancing was the only physical activity associated with a lower risk of dementia.[11] Similar results emerged from a 2012 study by researchers at North Dakota's Minot State University investigating the impact of the physical and expressive dimensions of dance on the brain functioning.[12] A small group of 35 seniors ages 65 to 91 from the community participated in Zumba or yoga classes for 30 minutes twice a week at a local dance studio.[13] Participants' cognition and processing skills were assessed using the Stroop test after six weeks and after 12 weeks.[14] The researchers found that dancing to Zumba significantly improves specific cognitive skills, such as visual recognition and decision-making as well as uplifting the moods of participants.[15] Researcher Terry Eckmann, who was "surprised to find that significant of a change," stated that her "Research suggests that freestyle partner dancing may offer the best benefit of all."[16] Further confirmation for the impacts of exercise on brain health came from another study by researchers at the University of Wisconsin School of Medicine and Public Health, whose findings were published in 2014.[17] The researchers who examined 317 late-middle-aged adults found that those who engaged in regular exercise at least five times a week displayed fewer of the age-related changes in the brain associated with Alzheimer's and performed better on memory, visual-spatial and cognitive tests.[18] In effect, those older adults who regularly exercised had less accumulation of beta-amyloid plaque, less shrinkage of the hippocampus, more effective glucose utilization in the brain, and fewer neurofibrillary tangles.[19] Thus, in a research report titled *Remember to Dance* that evaluated the impact of dance activities on people with dementia, Trish Vella-Burrows and Lian Wilson, concluded that dance is impactful because it "uniquely combine[s] thinking, feeling, sensing and doing. It has strong effects on physiological and psychological well-being, combining the benefits of physical exercise with heightened sensory awareness, cognitive function, creativity, inter-personal contact and emotional expression – a potent cocktail."[20] This report echoes the results of numerous studies that consistently link sustained physical activity with improved cognitive health, suggesting that preemptive lifestyle modifications may help stave off or perhaps even delay dementia. In effect, through the production of neurotransmitters, hormones, and growth factors, dance movement has significant neurological impacts, supporting brain health, and overall well-being. By making regular dancing a habit and hobby, Elizabeth, Erin, and Marigrace keep their brains more youthful and effectively acquire a protective effect against the dangers of neurodegenerative decline.[21]

*****

In a study published in *Frontiers in Human Neuroscience* in 2017, Kathrin Rehfeld and her colleagues assessed the impact of dancing versus participation in a "classical cardiovascular fitness program" among older adults (average age 68), focusing on the relative impact of these activities on "neuroplasticity" and the implications for dementia prevention.[22] Participants engaged in an 18-month weekly course during which they had to learn new, complex, and constantly changing dance routines in "a specially designed, sensorimotor, and cognitive challenging dance program in comparison to a classical cardiovascular fitness program."[23] The researchers introduced participants to different genres including, jazz, square dance, line dance, and various Latin-American dances, increasing the challenge by changing steps, arm-patterns, formations, speed, rhythms every second week. [24] Moreover, participants were expected to remember these dance routines under time pressure without help from the teacher.[25] Researchers stated they were especially focused on understanding the impact of these activities on the hippocampus for three reasons: (1) it is a brain structure that is "especially affected by normal and pathological aging;" (2) it performs a "key role in major cognitive processes...;" and, (3) it is "involved in keeping one's balance, a function which is crucial for well-being and quality of life." [26] The researchers found that while both dancing and fitness training "led to increases in hippocampal subfield volumes," the dancers exhibited hippocampal "volume increases in more subfields (four out of five)." [27] Moreover, they concluded "only dancing led to an increase in one subfield of the right" hippocampus called the subiculum. [28] The researchers also determined that "dancing was superior to standard fitness" with regard to postural control, "as expressed by a larger increase in the composite score of our balance test and improved use of all three sensory systems." [29] While acknowledging that both activities can increase hippocampal volume, only the dancers showed an increase in the dentate gyrus (DG) of the hippocampus - the area where adult neurogenesis occurs in animal studies.[30] Compared to traditional fitness workouts, "other factors inherent in dancing," specifically, the "sensorimotor demanding" nature of dance activity, including the extra mental challenges of learning complex and changing dances routines, may have given the dancers the edge in terms of hippocampal growth and anti-aging benefits.[31] They suggested the "sensory enrichment" and stimulation of dance activity could have caused the new neurons to survive and flourish. [32] Therefore, the researchers concluded, "the additional challenges involved in our dance program, namely cognitive and sensorimotor stimulation, induced extra HC volume changes in addition to those attributable to physical fitness alone." [33] The researchers theorized superior improvement in balance observed among dancers occurred because "dancing drives all three senses and presumably also improves the integration of sensorimotor, visual, and vestibular information."[34]

Likewise, in another study published in *PLOS 1* in 2018, Kathrin Rehfeld, once again, focused on the impact of dancing versus fitness training on adults aged 63–80 years, this time joined by researchers at the German Center for Neurodegenerative Diseases in Magdeburg University.[35] The researchers designed a challenging sixth-month program for 38 persons randomly assigned to a dance group or the control group; all participants underwent an elaborate pre-assessment related to factors such as cognition, memory, and fitness levels.[36] Under the supervision of a qualified dance instructor, dancers had to learn new and increasingly difficult choreographies of five different genres - line dance, jazz dance, rock 'n' roll, Latin-American dance, and square dance.[37] The program, which featured progressively complex lessons, emphasized continuous learning of new skills, movements, patterns, coordination as well as memorization of step sequences and accurate recall and execution of steps under time pressure. [38] An elaborate post-assessment was conducted emphasizing general cognition, attention, memory, balance, cardio-respiratory fitness, and BDNF levels. [39] The researchers found dancing led to a greater increase of gray matter in the brain than the conventional exercise program, especially areas associated with working and long-term memory, executive functions, cognitive control, and attention regulation. [40] Researchers observed a noticeable increase in gray matter in the temporal lobe area associated with episodic memory that typically deteriorates at the onset of Alzheimer's disease. In addition, they noticed more gray matter in the brain areas central to auditory short-term memory as well as audio-visual integration. [41] The researchers theorized these gray matter increases came about because dancing encompasses "multisensory stimulation with visual, sensory and auditory input." [42] Rehfeld and her colleagues also observed increases in white matter, particularly in the frontal and parietal lobes and especially regarding the expansion of the corpus callosum that connects nearly all parts of the hemispheres and ensures the communication between both cerebral hemispheres. [43] In effect, dancing can strengthen the links and interaction between both cerebral hemispheres – critical because, as we age, neurodegenerative decline in this area fuels cognitive impairments. [44] These results are especially promising from a preventive health perspective because they suggest proactive steps can be taken to protect cognitive functions typically threatened by age-related neurodegenerative decline.[45]

As always, the experiences of dancers themselves convey a vitality that research findings cannot match. One cannot help but be inspired by the lifelong passion that 75-year old Alice Simpson has for dancing. In a comment to the Post, Ms. Simpson wrote about how her enthusiasm for dance has positively impacted her health and well-being.[46] At age 75, when so many are sedentary, she is still going strong, very strong - regularly dancing to classic tango songs by the likes of

Astor Piazzolla, Carlos Gardel, and the Gotan Project

"three times a week, and would dance five if that was

possible."[47] Her sustained and consistent dancing has

improved her "balance, concentration, and focus…" and

she stated that she can "stand taller, move more easily,

smile more…"[48] Ms. Simpson also lauded the

importance of dancing as a way to experience a greater

feeling of social connectedness, including meeting "new

friends of all ages and plenty of hugs."[49] Well-schooled

on social etiquette of ballroom dance, she quoted from

W.P Hazard's "The Ballroom Companion," advising

dancers to "converse about music and the opera,

dancing and the ballet, concerts and the theater …" and

avoid controversial subjects, particularly "…religion and

politics, especially with a stranger."[50] She wrote the

ability to go out and "dance, dance, dance" enabled her

to re-connect with memories of the past such that for

the brief "minute and a half" dancing in her "partner's

arms," she was able to "remember what love was."[51] Like any consummate aficionado, she is still imbued by "a desire to improve" to learn new steps, welcoming the "exciting challenge at a time of life that doesn't always provide such."[52] Similarly, another lifelong practitioner (VKG), who started dancing at seven and is "still dancing," at age 70, penned a powerful testimonial to the power of dance as a healthful mind-body workout. [53] She shared that she has been "attending several dance classes each week" for over a decade at her local Y, under the auspices of an instructor "who changes the dances every 3-4 months."[54] She also added that "those of us who have been dancing all our lives know that it benefits our brains as much as our bodies... We have to learn the new choreography of many dances, a challenge to mind and body." [55] In addition, she reminded us that one is never too old to dance, with a deft critique of antiquated Victorian manuals that frowned upon dance by older women writing, "Most of us in the classes, including the instructor, are women "of a certain age."[56]

*****

Dancers like seventy-something-year-old Ms. Simpson are getting much more than physical exercise on the dance floor: dancing regularly turns out to be some of the most potent anti-aging medicine. In an article published in the *Frontiers of Aging in Neuroscience* in 2017, Agnieszka Burzynska and her colleagues examined the effects of lifestyle interventions such as complex country dances, walking, and nutrition on white matter integrity.[57] A supposedly normal side effect of aging is the deterioration or "structural disconnection" of cerebral white matter; this outcome typically undermines cognitive functions such as processing speed and accelerates neurodegenerative decline.[58] To better understand the impact of physical activity on aging, the researchers collected MRI imaging data from 174 healthy but low-active adults in their 60s and 70s and randomly assigned them to one of four lifestyle interventions for six months.[59] The researchers concluded the dancers' brains showed real improvement in white matter health - revealing denser white matter in the fornix. [60] This finding was auspicious because the fornix is the primary output track or efferent system of the hippocampus, vitally involved with processing speed, memory, and the capacity to absorb, analyze and react to new information.[61] The findings suggested physical activity slows white matter degeneration and that combining the physical and cognitive engagement of dance movement may be even more beneficial for white matter health.[62] The experiences of country dancers like William in Santa Barbara exemplify the potency of dance, reifying the above research findings.[63] An avid

contra dancer for about three decades, William attests

to contra's cognitive benefits, noting that participants

appreciate the complicated moves that test or challenge

dancers mentally, effectively providing both a brain and

body workout.[64] With intricate patterns that require

quick recall, focused concentration, and deft execution,

William shared that contra dancing keeps the "mind

stimulated" helping "people with active minds" attain

"ripe old ages."[65] He further shared that he has often

encountered "numerous dancers with science and math

backgrounds particularly attracted to contras with their

complex, but easily-learned movements."[66] Like many

other dancers eager to share their love of the genre,

William confirmed that one of the best things about

contra dancing is that it brings entire generations of

families out together to the dance floor, enabling warm

"social interaction [that] boosts endorphins."[67] He

shared that "over the years," he has "danced with several people in their 90's, as well as children as young as 2" because contra dancing is "a family-community form of dance."[68] The exciting cognitive and social benefits enjoyed by contra dancers in Santa Barbara were reportedly documented by NHK television for a Japanese science program.[69] The mental challenges of dance are by no means unique to contra dance as and can be experienced in various forms of dance experiences. For example, Lisa N. of Los Angeles shared that after she "started choreographed dance classes a few years ago, ...[she] was shocked at how hard it was... not because of the physical demands, (although those were substantial), but because of the mental demands."[70] An inveterate athlete who had been active in sports throughout her life, Lisa was surprised by the "memorization, the coordination, [and] the pace..." required in dancing. She conceded until she took up dancing, she had "never felt such a complete exercise. Better yet, it was fun."[71]

*****

Whether it takes the form of Zumba, contra dance, or yoga, movement is positively beneficial for health. In a study published in the *Journal of Alzheimer's Disease*, Harris Eyre and his colleagues investigated the link between performance on memory tests and resting-state functional connectivity before and after a yoga intervention.[72] Participants aged 55 and older with mild cognitive impairment were randomly assigned to receive either a yoga intervention or memory enhancement training (MET) for 12 weeks.[73] Resting-state functional connectivity was measured by MRIs to map correlations between brain networks and memory performance changes over time.[74] The yoga participants engaged in Kirtan Kriya yoga meditation that involves chanting a mantra, hand movements, and visualization, augmented with weekly Kundalini yoga classes.[75] Researchers found both the KK yoga intervention and MET were equally effective in improving memory functions and "functional connectivity," particularly in relation to verbal memory performance.[76] Moreover, participants who engaged in physical activity plus meditation outperformed the MET group in terms of enhanced moods and visuospatial memory - crucial for balance, depth perception, object recognition, and spatial navigation.[77] Researchers theorized the enhanced verbal and visuo-spatial memory performance might be attributable to the chanting mantra and meditation of KK yoga combined with visualization, effectively deepening awareness and turbo-charging specific verbal, visual, and spatial skills. [78] The researchers also theorized yoga's effect on the brain might also be linked to its impact on the following: reducing inflammation, lowering stress, increasing antioxidant levels, boosting telomerase activity, increasing BDNF levels, and enhancing neuroplasticity.[79] The study suggests combining mindfulness meditation and breathing exercises with yoga movement is a potent mix to combat neurodegenerative decline.[80]

In another study published in the *Journal of Alzheimer's Disease* in 2016, Cyrus Raji and colleagues used caloric expenditure as a proxy for physical activity to assess the corresponding impact on gray matter volume.[81] Of note, the study used the broad definition of physical activity as embraced by the revamped federal physical-activity guidelines that encourage people to be more mobile, regardless of the type of movement.[82] The UCLA researchers analyzed a subset of 876 normal and cognitively- impaired persons (mean age 78.3) recruited from the Cardiovascular Health Study - a multisite population-based longitudinal study of adults 65 and older.[83] The researchers examined participants' energy output conceived as kilocalories per week based on responses to lifestyle questionnaires. [84] Researchers also conducted cognitive assessments ranging from normal, mild to Alzheimer's as well as volumetric MRI brain scans. [85] The study showed higher energy expenditure from wide-ranging physical activities, including ballroom dancing, gardening, walking, jogging, and cycling, were linked to larger gray matter volumes in the elderly - notwithstanding cognitive status.[86] The top quartile of physically active participants with cognitive impairment at baseline showed substantially more gray matter in the brain's areas connected to memory and higher--level thinking – a sign of improved brain health.[87] There was a noticeable gray matter volume increase in the frontal, temporal, and parietal lobes, as well as the hippocampus, thalamus, and basal ganglia. [88] Consistent physical activity or high caloric expenditure also mitigated gray matter volume loss and neurodegeneration in other areas; participants whose physical activity increased over five years demonstrated even more pronounced increases in gray-matter volume.[89] The research further reaffirmed the link between high fitness levels and larger hippocampal volume, as exercise precipitates adult hippocampal neurogenesis, even in elderly participants. [90] The findings also confirmed that adults with larger hippocampal volumes perform better in short-term memory tests and have a reduced risk of developing Alzheimer's. [91] Overall, participants with a higher amount of gray matter associated with physical activity saw a 50% reduction in their risk of memory deterioration or Alzheimer's five years later.[92] It is not too late to start. Several other studies confirm the benefits of taking up dance even after the onset of mild cognitive impairment and/or late in life. For example, researchers in Greece found that older persons with mild cognitive impairment who engaged in ballroom dancing improved their thinking and memory after a 10-month-long ballroom dancing class.[93] Similarly, researchers at the University of Illinois at Chicago reported participants in a Latin ballroom dance program for older sedentary adults (BAILAMOS) reported improvements in memory, attention, and focus.[94]

When it comes to delaying or staving off dementia, long-term fitness buffs appear to have a strong advantage. In a study published in the *Journal of Neurology* in 2018, researchers tracked fitness levels of 191 middle-aged women who were part of a larger population health study of 1,462 Swedish women aged 38 - 60.[95]

Researchers assessed cardiovascular fitness levels as determined by the maximum performance on a stationary cycle machine before exhaustion; the stationary bikes were equipped with ergometers to assess work output and peak workload.[96] The researchers further subdivided the participants into three categories: low fitness - generating 80 watts; medium – generating 88 – 112 watts, and high fitness, generating 120 watts.[97] Analysis of data collected after a 44-year period showed a 32% incidence of dementia (19 of 59) in the low-fitness category and a 25% incidence of dementia (23 of 59) in the medium fitness category.[98] Among the high fitness group, only 5% (2 women) developed dementia; the fittest women at midlife were 88% less likely than the moderately fit peers to develop dementia.[99] While the least fit developed dementia at average age 81, the onset of dementia among the fittest was pushed back about nine years to age ninety; researchers adjusted results for age, height, triglyceride levels, hypertension, smoking, wine consumption, physical inactivity, and income.[100] Commenting on the study, Nicole Spartano of Boston University stated these results "suggest underlying poor cardiovascular health may partially explain the relationship between fitness and brain health." [101]

It is not too late: studies show that even sedentary late bloomers can reap substantial benefits from physical activity by turning over a new leaf and taking the first dance step towards brain health. In an article published in the *Journal of Applied Physiology, Nutrition, and Metabolism* in 2019, Ana Kovacevic and her colleagues examined the impact of aerobic exercise intensity on memory and general cognitive abilities of older adults in their sixties.[102] In the community-based study, researchers assessed participants' high-interference memory using a Mnemonic Similarity Task, which measures recall of similar memories, something that declines with age and could signal cognitive impairment.[103] Executive functions were assessed using Go/No-go and Flanker tasks.[104] Subsequently, participants were randomly assigned into three groups. (1) High-intensity interval (HIIT) treadmill walkers for four minutes who pushed their heart rate to 90% of their VO Max. (2) Treadmill walkers engaged in moderate continuous training (MCT) three times weekly for 50 minutes; and, (3) a control group of non-exercisers who merely stretched in the lab (CON).[105] When researchers re-tested the participants after 12 weeks, only the HIIT walkers showed substantial improvements in physical endurance and memory performance; and, "greater improvements in memory correlated with greater increases in fitness." [106] The findings suggest aerobic exercise programs could be a vital component in programs to "enhance memory in older adults," and even previously inactive participants who engage in "higher intensity exercise," can reap great rewards."[107] As researcher Jennifer Heisz at McMaster University stated, "it is not too late" for older people to begin exercise regimens to safeguard their memories, especially through higher intensity workouts that raise the heart rate.[108] Similarly, Norwegian researchers who looked at fitness levels over time and the risk of dementia found good news, even for late bloomers. In an article published in *The Lancet Public Health* in 2019, Atefe Tari and her colleagues reviewed records of 30,000 middle-aged persons from a study of adults in Norway's Trondheim region in the 1980s - categorizing them by fitness and relative variations over time.[109] Subsequently, researchers checked records from nursing homes and memory clinics to determine which participants developed dementia in a 20-year follow-up period and whether relative cardiovascular fitness reduced their risk of cognitive decline and impairment.[110] Researchers found participants with persistently high estimated cardiorespiratory fitness levels had a 40–50% reduced risk of incident dementia, a 30–40% reduced risk of dementia-related death, a 2-year delay in onset of dementia, and a 2 - 3-year increase in life expectancy.[111] The cake is not yet baked, at midlife or retirement age – just as long as you get going: similar results were observed among the late bloomers, those unfit at middle age but who subsequently enhanced their fitness levels. [112] As the study lead author Atefe Tari stated, since "there is currently no effective drug for dementia, it is important to focus on prevention. Exercise that improves fitness appears to be one of the best medicines to prevent dementia."[113] When next you read about the local dance studio offering tango classes, besides the opportunity to meet and socialize with interesting people, you have a chance to develop a habit that could potentially save you from cognitive and mobility impairments and even disability later in life.

*****

For people with Parkinson's or other conditions that limit motor function, dancing the tango is more than fun and games. Over the last past decade, there has been growing interest in understanding how dance impacts Parkinson's disease, especially apropos improving motor skills and patients' overall quality of life. Studies show sustained participation in dance interventions lessens the debilitating impacts of impairments endured by Parkinson's patients. Patients often experience demonstrably significant improvements in functional mobility, locomotion, balance, coordination, flexibility, general physical fitness, cognitive performance, mood, and overall quality of life. For example, in an article published in *Gait and Posture* in 2005, Patricia McKinley and her colleagues at McGill University set out to investigate the impact of Argentine tango dancing on balance and complex task performance in at-risk elderly.[114] Thirty elderly residents from Montreal's Cummings Jewish Senior Center, ages ranging from 62 to 90, were invited to participate in the study; albeit in good health, they had all fallen within the previous year and had developed a fear of falls.[115] For ten weeks, one half of the group danced away in tango classes while the control group was assigned to walk. [116] After ten weeks of lessons, researchers found the tango dancers exhibited remarkable improvements in gait, balance, posture, and motor coordination, including moving in confined spaces.[117] Researchers also found the tango boosted cognitive capacities and was more effective for multitasking and enhancing the performance of complex tasks, such as navigating restricted spaces without stumbling and falling.[118] Meanwhile, in another article published in 2007 in *Journal of Neurologic Physical Therapy,* Madeleine Hackney and Gammon Earhart assessed the effectiveness of tango dancing versus traditional exercise on improving functional mobility deficits in persons with Parkinson's Disease.[119] After nineteen participants, randomly assigned to a tango group, or a group exercise class, completed a 20-week program, a subsequent evaluation revealed only the tango group showed significant improvements on the Berg Balance Scale.[120] Unlike the exercise group, the tango group also improved on the Timed Up and Go test.[121]

Over a decade ago, Lisa Heiberger and her fellow neuroscientists teamed up to host an 8-month weekly

dance class in Freiburg, Germany, with dance
instructors who had expertise in ballet, jazz steps,
contemporary dance, dance theater, and-improvisation.
[122] Featuring dances by famous choreographers, the
program was also modeled after the course offered by
Mark Morris Dance Group/Brooklyn Parkinson Group,
with movement sequences that combined elements of
ballet, jazz steps, contemporary dance, and dance
theater.[123] Classical ballet sequences were chosen for
their "versatile aspects that lead to a better body-feeling
and –awareness," and because the ballet requires "grace
and elegance" that also heighten "esthetic perception.
[124] Moreover, ballet performance also enhances balance
(from increased body tension), flexibility, posture,
muscle strength, coordination, and proprioceptive
acuity.[125] Jazz sequences with rhythms performed to a
consistent and "predictable beat" were used to facilitate
"rhythmic walking steps;" meanwhile, contemporary

dance music, including modern dance and improvisation, was used to facilitate a more "conscious and more natural" dance with an "easy flow of energy." [126] Dance theater sequences were also chosen because they often rely on techniques such as facial expressions, pantomime, speech, everyday movements/gestures, and self-produced noises to communicate feelings, tell stories or share experiences. [127] Participants began with a warmup comprised of physical and mental dance exercises "to produce an optimal psycho-physical constitution" for performance and practiced with "one hand touching at the barre to refine proprioception and enhance balance. [128] Dance exercises were "executed without tactile feedback" and choreographed sequences were performed under the guidance of the teacher; class ended with a bowing "la reverence," akin to traditional ballet but now "integrated to the farewell in a standing circle holding hands." [129]

In an article published in *Frontiers in Aging Neuroscience* in 2011, Lisa Heiberger and her colleagues shared the results of this 8-month weekly dance intervention in Freiburg on the motor control of PD patients as well as the impact on the quality of life of patients and their caregivers.[130] The researchers concluded the weekly ballet dance classes had a beneficial effect on the functional mobility of individuals with PD, including "immediate positive effects on motor deficits, especially on the rigidity of the limbs as well as on fine motor skills and facial expression." [131] The classes helped "activate the patients" substantially, demonstrating dance is "a very efficient activity to improve mobility and well-being." [132] There were overall positive impacts on social life, health, body-feeling, and daily competences; there were also significant short-term improvements in rigidity scores,

hand movements, finger taps, and facial expression.[133]
In addition, researchers showed that the quality of life
of the patients and their caregivers improved in tandem
over the 8-month regimen, and they concluded that
compared to other exercise interventions, dancing "may
lead to better therapeutic strategies as it is engaging
and enjoyable." [134]   The limits of the research design did
not enable researchers to conclude whether the dance
program's physical or social aspects precipitated the
positive improvements. Immediately after the dance
class, 8 out of 11 patients reported improvement of
their body-feeling; 9 out of 11 reported an improved
"state of mind;" after the dance class. [135]   In addition, 7
out of 11 patients reported the "consequences of the
dance class" positively impacted their daily quality of
life, some for a few hours and others for several days;
10 of 11 patients reported an improvement of their
mobility, half stating, it improved "a little bit" and the

others noting "mobility improved a lot." [136] In written feedback, patients captured their improvement in vivid ways reflecting their increased flexibility and joy as they experienced movement in a welcoming social setting.[137] One patient exulted: "The rhythm. I want to fly. It gives me a swinging feeling. I feel relaxed after the dance lesson. Before, I'm always very stiff." [138] Another stated, "…Dancing gives me a good feeling. It liberates me."[139] Several others valued the feeling of "togetherness" and the "social contacts" afforded by the experience, especially as a distraction from focusing on the disease - with one patient summing it up thusly: "It feels good to be with many people. Otherwise, I live in isolation." [140] Several comments attested to the "fun and joy" of the dance class, one person calling it "the highlight of the week" while another stated: "The dance lesson is very important to me. It is a pleasure. Should take place more often. It makes me feel incredibly good and helps me to forget my illness." [141] Beyond the applied tests, videos of the classes also portrayed more vividly the "large amount of motor learning" accomplished. [142] Patients can be seen making moves they could not make at the doctor's offices, often exceeding the outcomes at traditional physical therapies and rehabilitation programs. [143]

In a rejoinder of sorts to an earlier article she co-authored in 2007 in the *Journal of Neurologic Physical Therapy*, Gammon Earhart teamed up with Ryan Duncan to further investigate the impact of the tango on PD. In an article published in *The Journal of Alternative and Complementary Medicine* in 2014, Duncan and Earhart investigated the effects of sustained participation in a community-based tango dance class on Parkinson's symptoms.[144] In a randomized controlled trial, ten participants, in their mid to late sixties, were assigned either to an Argentine Tango dance group or a control group.[145] The dancing group was assigned to a community-based Argentine tango class for one hour twice weekly for two years while the control group was left to their own devices. [146] Researchers conducted blinded assessments of key measures related to disease severity and functional mobility, first at baseline, then subsequently at 12 and 24 months. [147] The researchers concluded the dancers' participation in the sustained community-based therapeutic tango intervention "was associated with improvements in motor and non-motor symptom severity, performance on activities of daily living, and balance." [148] Unlike the control group, dancers experienced less severe PD symptoms, and improvements in balance, gait velocity, and functional mobility, particularly "noteworthy given the progressive nature of PD."[149] Researchers maintained tango is well-suited for dance therapy because dancers walk to-and-fro in structured rhythmic patterns while performing sequences of intricate steps with taut-muscled movements that engage working memory. [150] Tango dancers maintain focus, processing multiple inputs and outputs, including maintaining eye contact with their dance partner and being mindful of their environment.[151] The perception of tango as the go-to dance for therapeutic interventions was further reinforced after the announcement of findings from another research project, this time a collaboration between researchers at the Montreal Neurological Institute and Hospital -The Neuro, McGill University, and the Research Institute of the McGill University Health Centre. In an article published in *Complementary Therapies in Medicine* in 2015, Silvia Romenets and her colleagues undertook a randomized control study to investigate the effectiveness of tango as a complementary therapy for motor and non-motor manifestations in PD.[152] In the first major effort to assess the impact of the tango on motor symptoms (balance and functional mobility) as well as non-motor symptoms (satisfaction, quality of life), 40 male and female participants with idiopathic Parkinson's disease from the Movement disorder clinic and dance studio at McGill University Health Center were selected for the 12-week study, divided into two randomized groups.[153] Under the guidance of two professional dance teachers, the first group of 24 patients participated in partnered tango classes in dance studios; the control group engaged in self-directed exercise.[154] The researchers found dancing the tango can result in improved balance and "functional mobility" in patients with Parkinson's, noting also that tango dancers demonstrated a "borderline improvement in walk with pivot turns;" tango dancing also resulted in "modest benefits" in improved cognition. [155]   While researchers observed Mini-BESTest improvement in the tango group compared to control, they noted this finding needed further confirmation in longer-term trials "explicitly powered for cognition." [156]   Researchers also found the tango dancers experienced a lessening of fatigue and an "overall" increase in treatment satisfaction, especially regarding the positive impact of socialization. [157]   Study lead author, Dr. Silvia Rios Romenets, stated, "the tango was helpful in significantly improving balance and functional mobility, and seemed to encourage patients to appreciate their general course of therapy." [158] She also noted these results were consistent with the "accumulating evidence that habitual physical activity is associated with a lower risk of developing PD, which suggests a potential slowing of PD progression." [159]

There is growing evidence that tai chi practice can also enhance the strength, flexibility, and cognitive performance of Parkinson's patients, thereby reducing their susceptibility to falls. With its focus on mindful movement, Tai chi is effectively what Peter Wayne at Brigham and Women's Hospital calls a more ritualized and structured form of dance.[160] Wayne, who is conducting clinical trials on patients with balance disorders, contends tai chi may be particularly appropriate for these patients.[161] Tai chi is a viable complementary therapy because the immersion in mindful movement could achieve a more efficient mind-body nexus that helps PD patients overcome motor disabilities and age-related neurodegenerative decline.[162] In an article published in the *New England Journal of Medicine,* Fuzhong Li and his colleagues conducted a randomized, controlled trial to determine whether "a tailored tai chi program could improve postural control in patients with idiopathic Parkinson's disease."[163] The researchers randomly assigned 195 patients to engage in 60-minute exercise sessions twice weekly for 24 weeks, assigning them to either tai chi, resistance training, or stretching.[164] The patients were all in stage 1 - 4 of the disease on the Hoehn and Yahr staging scale (5 being the most severe disease). [165] Primary outcomes centered on postural stability (maximum excursion and directional control), while secondary motor outcomes including gait, strength, and number of falls. [166] Researchers found the tai chi group consistently outperformed the resistance-training and stretching groups regarding primary outcomes and also outperformed the stretching group in all secondary outcomes. [167] Tai chi did better than the resistance-training group in stride length and functional reach; tai chi also reduced the incidence of falls compared with stretching but not as compared with resistance training.

[168] Overall, tai chi patients were physically stronger, had fewer balance impairments, and exhibited slower rates of decline in general motor control; these beneficial impacts persisted for up to 3 months after the intervention. [169] The researchers concluded that for patients with mild-to-moderate Parkinson's disease, tai chi training enhances "functional capacity," improves balance, and reduces falls. [170]

Since 2010, the University of Roehampton has partnered with the English National Ballet to explore and document dancers' experience with PD, focusing on outcomes such as functional mobility, social engagement, dancers' experiences, and overall quality of life. [171] Led by Drs. Sara Houston and Ashley McGill, the study tracks participants' progress using observation, biomedical measurements, clinical rating scales, one-on-one interviews, focus groups, questionnaires, participant diaries, and film footage. [172] Results are measured against a control group of non-dancers with PD.[173] In 2014 the researchers published findings revealing dancers experience "a physically and socially-active lifestyle" because the program provides "a community of support" that helps them "stay motivated and maintain or improve other non-motor aspects of daily life." [174] They also found dancing with PD "encourages a feeling of capability, aiding fluency of movement, postural stability, and decreases the amount of temporary freezing, despite progression of disease." [175] While **PD can cause muscles to** "stiffen up very easily," **the researchers found regular dancing lessens rigidity of movements, improves** "muscle tone" **and** "keeps **muscles loose," enabling the dancers to** "get used to dealing with balancing and moving in different ways." [176] **The researchers also found that dancing clearly** "improved quality of life" and was a "positive experience" that helped the patients "support each other" and stay "focused on dancing and not on the disease." [177] Patients' feedback, as documented in the report, describes elation and pride as some go from struggling to take a few steps to dancing and enjoying themselves with more fluid motions.[178] Patients also describe the positive psychological and social benefits, including increased confidence, an overall increase in life satisfaction, and general well-being.[179] For example, several participants commented on the challenging nature of the mental workouts which one dancer described as "liberation and refreshing" and yet another as "taxing on the memory and that is what is brilliant." [180] The progress reportedly surprised many healthcare professionals who gained a new appreciation of dance as a therapeutic intervention.[181]

Overall, for patients with Parkinson's, researchers are finding dancing seems to result in better outcomes than conventional exercise. Researchers find it reassuring that PD patients persist and positively engage with their prescribed dance regimens, especially when compared to regular exercise programs, which many find uninviting and uninspiring. [182] Such relatively high persistence levels are particularly significant because over 50 percent of patients with Parkinson's do not fulfill the minimum weekly exercise recommendations.[183]   However, it appears that dancing inspires Parkinson's patients to get up and move despite the challenges they face. Researchers suggest positive social engagement, social support structure, and uplifted moods resulting from dance classes may enhance the overall experience and promote sustained compliance with dance regimens. [184] It is thought dance classes help counter some of the negative cognitive and emotional impacts patients

experience, perhaps even lessening depression and

anxiety symptoms.[185] Patricia McKinley, who has

conducted several major studies on the subject, believes

that dancing is ideal for an older population that is not

often attracted to traditional exercise. [186] She thinks

dance overcomes the usual reasons for not exercising

because it is "fun, it's a group activity, and it has a

tangible goal that can be perceived not only by the

dancer, but [also] by his or her family and friends."[187]

Moreover, Dr. Dominguez, a neurologist in the

Philippines, maintains there is a "physiologic,

morphologic and anatomic basis" for the observed

outcomes on dance, even more so than other exercises

because dance involves more mindful and purposeful

learning along with the helping power of music.[188]

Dance classes also provide a safe, comfortable, non-

judgmental, and enjoyable space, helping to mitigate the

common tendency to withdraw, become more isolated, and experience greater loneliness.[189] As Dr. Bronte-Stewart at Stanford stated, dancing provides patients an opportunity "to do something beautiful and graceful" and be part of a welcoming community, with many reporting they feel "less helpless" and attesting to numerous "physical, emotional, and social benefits."[190] Since dance for Parkinson's classes are designed to engage multiple senses, foster creative expression, and energize social interaction, participants find the experiences inspiring and are highly motivated to attend consistently. [191] Patients' testimonials often allude to the joy they experience in these programs, particularly the uplifting combination of music, dancing and engaging company, as well as the much-needed distraction that these events provide, especially compared to the grind of mere 'exercise.'[192] Patients often indicate they enjoy participating because the dance programs offer an opportunity to fend off the loneliness and depression often associated with neurological disorders. [193] During such positive therapeutic interventions, patients report they forget about the illness, and can briefly relax and have a little fun while they dance to great music with friends, partners, or companions in uplifting social settings. [194] At the Stanford PD program, Albert Cohen, 87, enjoyed the warm, caring, and "very beneficial" experience noting, "The attitude there is positive and receptive, which is worth a lot... I'm not sitting in a room doing nothing." [195] His wife, Betty, who attended the classes, is also buoyed by the social and emotional benefits of being a dancing partner as well as a "co-learner," noting the experience helps her come to terms with the very challenging situation. [196] Similarly, Ann Anderson, a patient taking a dance class for Parkinson's (Simply Ballroom) in Virginia, stated that dancing ballet at the studio was "the happiest day of the week." [197]   During

her ballet class, she was able to briefly transcend the

"very depressing, terrible disease," because as she put

it, "I'm always well when I come here."[198]   For example,

Victor Liu a 71-year old Virginia resident who attended

Simply Ballroom, a free dance class for Parkinson's

patients, stated dancing provided a reprieve from his

symptoms, noting: "I cannot walk, but I can dance."[199]

For sustained benefits, consistency and stick-to-

itiveness are critical.. Dr. Bronte-Stewart at Stanford

emphasizes the necessity to "keep training" the motor

system and the brain - to continue "movement in a

disease that otherwise limits movement, counteracting

the stiffness and slowness that the brain wants to

impart on the musculoskeletal system."[200] She

maintains that "training the machine" through exercise,

dance, and balance training will improve patients' "core

strength" and mitigate some of the undesirable motor

impacts of PD, like difficulty getting out of chairs or a car.[201] While the combination of rhythmic movement, exercise, and dance will certainly not cure dementia, Alzheimer's, and Parkinson's, it is one of the best ways to nourish and vitalize the brain so as to forestall or perhaps limit certain types of neurodegenerative decline. To be sure, there are always those who would like to see more scientific research to explain the positive outcomes experienced by patients with dementia, Alzheimer's, or Parkinson's who undergo dance interventions. Nonetheless, it is becoming increasingly difficult for skeptics to ignore the volume of research confirming the positive outcomes of dance and movement therapy as well as the consistent statements from patients attesting to their experiences.[202]

*****

Underlying findings regarding the neurological impact of dance movement are key assumptions about how dancing revitalizes and even reshapes the brain, strengthening the dynamism of new neuronal connections and enhancing neuroplasticity. As a physical and mental activity, dancing fosters an "enriched environment" where neurotrophines such as BDNF alter specific brain regions, foster neuroplasticity, and significantly improve cognitive function.[203] The manifold dance moves, the recollection of patterns and steps, the constant shifts of balance as well as the regular twists and turns, all engage the working memory and precipitate significant biochemical changes that boost hippocampal volume, nourish the brain environment and enhance functioning.[204] In an article published in *PLOS One* in 2018, Kathrin Rehfeld and her colleagues theorized dancing induced and accelerated adult hippocampal neurogenesis – the process whereby neural progenitor cells generate new neurons and increase connectivity in the hippocampus.[205] Unlike many temporary changes in the brain, researchers think new brain cells survive, even after one stops exercising because rejuvenating the hippocampus helps forestall age-related neurodegenerative decline and ailments such as Alzheimer's.[206] As Dr. Bronte-Stewart at Stanford observed, animal studies suggest a biological rationale for the enhanced neurologic function observed in people participating in dance interventions.[207] Studies show animals performing physical activity they enjoy can "regenerate adult stem cells" that can, in turn, help build muscle and other tissues, suggesting that "dance possibly may improve the brain's regeneration of its own stem cells."[208] Moreover, the studies showed those animals also experienced less inflammation - which may also help fight disease.[209]

Researchers theorize dancing has an even more profound impact on long-term brain health than plain vanilla exercise because of the lightning communication dancing instigates across multiple brain regions, and their intense engagement in diverse but inextricably related tasks.[210] Dancing to music engages multiple senses, including "auditory, visual and sensory stimulation" and impacts memory, motor learning, emotional perception, expression, interaction, mood, and overall health.[211] The effort is mentally exhilarating: the dancer recalls or learns new dances, reacts to rhythmic changes and novel patterns, and coordinates body movements, including using different body parts for different rhythms, not to mention striking a pose and keeping poise.[212] As Kathrin Rehfeld and her colleagues observed, the dancing brain is further challenged by variations in rhythm, including tempo, the "dynamic and temporal variability in the execution of partial (segmented) and whole-body movements."[213] The pairing of dance with music is a potent healing cocktail to sustain brain health and reduce premature neurodegenerative decline. As several studies above demonstrated, the music makes a difference. Rhythmic movement to music affects certain neuro-mechanisms in unusual but efficacious ways, creating what Krakauer termed the "pleasure double play," [214] as well as a dopamine fix, with significant ramifications for mood as well as healing. Music has been shown to help stroke and Parkinson's patients improve their gait or even resume walking as music helps stimulate brain regions that control movement.[215] Researchers have also found that "musical perception provokes visualization that influences the immune system," which benefits the brain.[216] Daniel Tarsy of the Parkinson's Center in Boston observed that when PD patients dance, the music stimulates the brain's emotional regions, perhaps helping bypass damaged brain cells, making movement easier. [217] Similarly, Robert Stern, a neurologist at Boston University, observed that dance and music most likely "get through to the person with Alzheimer's by exploiting the areas of the brain which are least impaired," forging a connection that "can have a profound impact."[218]

Improvisational dancing, with its lickety-split-second spontaneity and extemporaneous creativity, is likewise beneficial. It also involves processing auditory inputs, generating simultaneous motor outputs, engaging with rhythmic patterns while also recalling specific choreographic steps in sync with the music, rocking, and rolling while maintaining balance.[219] A dancer named Lisa described the subtle challenges entailed in spontaneously anticipating, following, and adjusting to rapidly changing cues from one's partner during social salsa dancing.[220] She wrote that the interaction could be both challenging and enthralling because "as a female follower.... you never know what the different male partners you dance with will throw at you."[221] In a situation that demands a heightened level of spontaneous ingenuity, the "follower" needs to be "able to interpret and develop a 'response' to the male's lead, in a split second."[222] Without missing a beat, the "follower either has to guess or else just 'create' her own follow, while also calculating how long of a follow or step/routine she can do, before anticipating ... another signal or lead."[223] She concluded that "The fact that this is all handled by the followers within milliseconds, is really quite fascinating."[224] And as Ginger Rodgers will add, all the more captivating when you do it backwards and on heels!

In effect, the intense mental gymnastics entailed in dance engage multiple brain regions, activate short-term memory, and reinforce the mind-body nexus vital to brain health. The stimulating impact of dance on the brain triggers new neuronal interconnections, re-wires brain circuitry, creates new brain cells, activates new receptors, and forges new pathways.[225] These impacts intensify synaptic density - the number of functional synapses that fire in a given brain area: higher synaptic density reflects more efficacious signal transmission in the brain and is considered a key indicator of brain health. [226] As Ericka P. Simpson, a neurologist at Houston's Methodist Hospital stated, challenging the brain with "new skills and new ways of doing things" increases connections in the brain, creates new pathways and expands synaptic density.[227] Therefore, Emily Cross and Luca Ticini suggest professional dancers, who routinely activate neural networks in dance as they deftly execute or replicate complex movements, display an extraordinary degree of plasticity between diverse brain regions and subcortical nuclei.[228] Dr. Edward Taub, a behavioral neuroscientist at the University of Alabama, contends the brain's "enormous plasticity" means 100% of the brain is available for use, with regions being deployed gaining strength at others' expense.[229] In effect, a new challenge, such as encouraging a stroke patient to use a damaged limb during dance therapy, can propel the brain to devise new pathways and re-wire or re-route. [230] Moreover, as discussed above, dancing slows the progression of neurodegenerative disorders like PD because movement triggers new neuronal firings and enhances neuroplasticity. The subsequent development of new and stronger connections in different parts of the brain could reduce the disjoints in communication between the brain and the CNS. [231] Thus, Dr. Joseph

Coyle at Harvard Medical suggested the positive outcomes observed in dance interventions arise from the brain's remarkable neuroplasticity as the cerebral cortex and hippocampus re-wire to create new neural pathways.[232]

In effect, for patients with neurodegenerative disorders, the unique attributes of dance make it an unusually potent medicine for stimulating the brain and perhaps even slowing its precipitous decline. Dr. Bronte -Stewart observed that patients afflicted with disorders such as Parkinson's benefit from the mental training involved in dance because they are "planning, using their executive function and ... sequencing, ... all frontal-lobe functions that can be impaired in Parkinson's."[233] Likewise, Joe Verghese thinks dancing has a protective effect because it "involves precise physical activity, listening to the music, remembering dance steps and taking your partner into account which is very mentally testing."[234]

Moreover, Dr. Tiffany Chow, a neurologist at Toronto's
Baycrest Center, thinks dancing to music helps
Parkinson's patients by instigating movement via
alternative portals in the brain, sidestepping the
pathways compromised by the disabling lack of
dopamine.[235] Since dancing can even engage and
stimulate different brain networks, some patients with
Parkinson's disease can dance even while unable to
walk. In effect, even while neuronal networks
implicated in walking are compromised by the disease,
dancing to music can trigger neuronal firings in other
areas that remain relatively unscathed.[236] As
neurologist Harry Kerasidis maintained, dancing
challenges even the injured brain to function in many
different ways, including synchronizing movement to
music, sequencing steps, and processing visual
signals.[237]

The studies above provide strong support for dance as a potent mental 'workout' that should be a key part of preventive health initiatives to combat neurodegenerative disorders. More than just a physical regimen, dancing engages mind, body and soul in a dynamic interplay of emotion, concentration, recall, learning, memorization, and execution of complex choreography in sync with the music, while maintaining poise and actively engaging with one's environment. These neurological impacts of dance movement and music sometimes come as a surprise even to patients who experience the power of 'dance medicine' for the first time. For example, several participants in the English National Ballet's Dance for Parkinson's collaboration with the University of Roehampton marveled at the cognitive aspects of dancing and the concentration required. [238] As one dancer stated, "Having to remember the next step as well as doing the bit before that is very difficult, it's good training really. And doing two things together..."[239] Another added, "It's the combination of movements, something which reactivates our brains."[240] The mental effort and significant brain stimulation in such dance interventions are also catalyzed by the increased social engagement among dancers, contributing to improved moods and the relative abatement in neurodegenerative decline.[241]

We have come a long way since very little was known about the neurological effects of dance movement. Scientists are now more aware of the powerful medicinal impacts of dance, arising from the brain's intense mental engagement and lightning-fast decision making, as the dancer plans, recalls, adapts, and seamlessly executes multiple choreographic and social tasks. Although dance is not a cure, there is a growing understanding that dancing is good for the brain because dance movement can foster the development of new neural pathways that enhance working memory and overall cognitive functioning.[242] Researchers think these neurological impacts help dancers develop "greater cognitive reserve and increased complexity of neuronal synapses" – attributes that have a protective effect against dementia and other neurodegenerative disorders.[243] It is often said 'use it or lose it,' and that appears to be the case here. According to Dr. Daniel Amen, the famous psychiatrist, people can improve brain health by learning new things, engaging in purposeful cognitive training, breaking routines, performing different tasks, cultivating new and stimulating friends, and various physical and mental exercises with an emphasis on novelty.[244] A culture of lifelong dancing and learning new dances in diverse and stimulating social settings is precisely what the doctor ordered for long-term brain health, including reducing

your risk of dementia and other age-related

neurodegenerative diseases. Even better, this "potent

cocktail" for preventing or delaying neurodegenerative

decline is virtually accessible to all and can be had on

the cheap, with no side effects.[245] As Vincent Fortanasce,

neurologist and author of "The Anti-Alzheimer's

Prescription" declared, "dancing is excellent for the

brain and body."[246] Indeed. Likewise, at the Weil

Cornell Medical Center, Dr. Richard Isaacson

recommends dancing to music as one of several

prophylactic lifestyle modifications that can stimulate

and nourish the brain and prevent Alzheimer's.[247]

IV. Healing Dance of the "Athletes of God"

Contemporary developments in dance science, including mounting evidence of the effectiveness of dance interventions in healthcare, are prompting health and medical professionals to rethink the therapeutic potential of dance. In addition to looking at the medicinal uses of dance movement today and the implications for dementia, Alzheimer's, and Parkinson's treatment, it is helpful to get a broader perspective on dance as a healing art. In some ways, the growing interest in dance and movement therapy is a case of 'back to the future,' as some look to the healing arts to find answers to contemporary healthcare challenges. In many societies, music, singing, and dance were central components of dance rituals for health, healing, and good fortune - ceremonies that were typically communal affairs. Understanding how many ancient societies apotheosized dance, and elevated it to a sacred art, provides useful historical context, particularly since even today, many describe the health benefits of dance as akin to a 'miracle.' Moreover, the psychological and social benefits of dance are congruent with its historical and sociological function through the ages as the glue that forged community and connectedness by cementing social bonds and deepening kinship.[1] Also, with its origins in what Lucian called "the mysteries" at the origins, the history of sacred dance also reifies the union of mind-body-spirit that is so aptly reflected in Albert Einstein's canonization of dancers as "the athletes of God."[2] As you will no doubt discover, the story of dance as a healing art is a story of our civilizational journey, an epic straddling the realms of history, anthropology, evolutionary biology, neuroscience, and religion, to name a few.

The healing art of dance has a pedigree that harkens back to dancing priests in ancient Egyptian temples to a diverse assortment of singing and dancing medicine men and women through the ages, including shamans, witchdoctors, and other healers. Dutch psychoanalyst, Joost Meerloo wrote, "the dance of the medicine man, priest or shaman belongs to the oldest form of medicine and psychotherapy in which the common exaltation and release of tensions [were] able to change man's physical and mental suffering..." [3] Historians have found significant evidence of ritual dance practices among the ancient civilizations of Sumerians, India, and Egypt. The ancient Sumerians, who developed instruments such as pipes, lyres, harps, and drums over 5000 years ago, had a robust ritual dance culture that they bequeathed to successor civilizations.[4] Some of the earliest records of organized dance rituals depict sacred dances in honor of Sumerian deities such as Madduk and extravagant

spring celebrations in honor of Ashtoreth, the goddess

of fertility.[5] Sumerian dance culture had a powerful

influence on the dances of the Babylonians, the

Assyrians even the much developed Egyptian

civilization.[6] Archaeologists have discovered several

extraordinary items from ancient Egypt, including a

wall painting featuring rattling harvest dances of Tomb

15 at Giza circa 2700 B.C.[7] Likewise, frescoes from

Tomb 113 at Thebes portray an African woman

adorned with vines doing a whirl dance.[8] Meanwhile,

on a wall painting of the 12th Dynasty of the Middle

Kingdom at Beni Hassan (Southern Egypt), artists

depicted three female dancers doing a pantomime titled

"The Wind" (c. 1900 B.C.).[9] Egypt is considered "the

birthplace of Western civilized dancing," because many

ritual dance conventions related to healing, birth,

harvest, and death can be traced to ancient Egypt.[10] For

example, the ancient Egyptians had extravagant ritual dance festivals to honor their gods, such as Hathor, the goddess of beauty, music, dancing, and the goddess Isis who, along with her brother-husband, Osiris, and her son Horus, constituted the seminal Abydos Triad.[11] Isis, considered "Mother of the Gods," introduced dancing to Egyptians, and people across the land were encouraged to visit her numerous temples and to pay homage through various rituals.[12] These dance ceremonies to seek good fortune, including health and well-being, were officiated by physician-priests who sang their medical scriptures at grand temples in solemn tones.[13] One of the most significant events in the Egyptian dance calendar was the festival of Abydos that celebrated the dancing god Osiris's resurrection - a commemoration very reminiscent of the festivities celebrating the Sumerian goddess, Ashtoreth.[14]   Believing the stars and planets were also doing cosmic dances in a "dancing universe," Egyptian astronomer priests also performed a secret Dance of the Stars, based on imitating the astral movements of celestial bodies. [15] In a circle dance, priests moved around an altar signifying the Sun, making zodiac signs and intoning rites as they danced from east to west, representing the movements of the heavenly bodies.[16] Besides the highly ceremonial ritual dances, the popular acrobatic dance traditions of ancient Egyptians strongly influenced developments in Crete that, in turn, became the source of Greek ritual dance traditions such as the dance of the Curetes.[17] Incidentally, the association of Egyptian dance with the physicality of acrobatics is hardly surprising since the early Egyptian word for dance also designated gymnastic exercises.[18]

As the evidence from these early civilizations showed, ritual dance was often inextricably linked with the sacred or the spiritual realm, where deities who created

dance were themselves, choreographers, and dancers.

History tells us dancing deities with healing powers

held sway over ancient peoples in many societies - a

phenomenon manifested in diverse accounts of the

creation. In a most elaborate myth featuring the great

Hindu Lord Shiva of the Sanskrit Rig Veda, the creation

of the universe was a ferociously spectacular "dance of

gods."[19] The twirling of this deity amidst a dust storm

of bedlam directed animating waves of enlivening

sound through matter, sparking it to life from a state of

inertia.[20] Through world-spawning moves involving

energy, force, dynamism, and vertiginous flow, Shiva

Nataraja concocts life itself, effectively causing the bang

that conjures up and manifests everything in the

universe. [21] Energized by rhythmic musicality, the

dance of creation is the articulated power through

which the life-force reveals itself and Shiva who "dances

and undances the cosmos" is at once "container and contained," encompassing totality and giving rise to a situation in which "the universe itself [is] pirouetting and dancing."[22] In this dance at the genesis, the elements of the creation are animated by Shiva, and matter itself is dancing and whirling, engrossing the ether that suffuses everything.[23] Lord Shiva, the first choreographer, dancer, and healer, "the master of both poison and medicine," enlivens the "manifold phenomena of the universe..." effectively undertaking a five-fold project: world creation, world preservation, world destruction, world incarnation (or illusive veiling) and world salvation (or release).[24]

With striking similarities, other creation mythologies from around the world also featured variants of dancing deities possessing other-worldly powers, including the supreme ability to heal. For example, among the Yoruba of West Africa, Oya, the mother goddess of fertility with Shiva-like prowess, is considered the incarnation of the dance of creation, simultaneously a mix of creator and destroyer, capable of invoking ferocious storms and the spirits of the deceased.[25] Among many Native American peoples, the Hoop Dance is considered a healing ceremony that helps restore harmony and equilibrium to the world.[26] The dance arose after the Creator gave a dying man a hoop with the understanding that every hoop danced into existence would create another – triggering a process that revived the man and spawned a world of living things.[27] In another account, the Jicarilla Apache Indians maintained the god-creator made a bird from mud and whirled it around in a dance, resulting in the production of dream-like forms; as the bird became dizzy from this twirling dance, images sprung out all around.[28] Meanwhile, according to the Mayan creation legend, the Popul Vuh, hero twins who returned from death at the hands of Xibalbans, traveled about using magic dances to outwit and overcome the Lords of Death. [29] Eventually, they succeeded in reviving their father, the Maize God - thereby enabling others to resurrect loved ones.[30] Similarly, in Japanese mythology, Amaterasu, the goddess of the sun and fields, withdrew into a cave after being insulted, plunging the world into total darkness.[31] When a council of the gods selected goddess Amano-Uzume to resolve the situation, she opted for the rather unusual approach of doing a dance on a bathtub turned upside down with her private parts exposed, prompting laughter from the gods. [32] Curious to find out what was going on, Amaterasu came out of the cave whose entrance was promptly sealed, thus restoring light to the world. [33] Even after thousands of years, the notion of a dancing deity with healing powers, reminiscent Shiva and early gnostic gospels, continues to resonate in popular culture. Recall the success of the mega-hit Irish musical "Lord of the Dance," that was inspired by Sydney Carter's 1963 song of the same name. As choreographer and dancer, Michael Flatley, flatly proclaimed, "I came down from heaven, and I danced on the earth ... I danced on the Sabbath, and I cured the lame ... I am the lord of the dance ..."[34]

In ancient Greek mythology, dance was not just a gift of the gods; it was central to the creation of the world itself. According to a creation myth told by the Pelasgians (Greek forerunners), after the Greek goddess Eurynome emerged from chaos, she performed a dance that brought about the separation of water and the sky.[35] Later, as Eurynome continued to dance on water, she stirred up wind and birthed an enormous serpent named Ophion.[36] Eventually, Eurynome morphs into a dove that produced a cosmic egg fertilized by Ophion, resulting in the heavens and earth and all within.[37] In a world where the gods were often depicted as dancers, the Greek pantheon of dancing gods including Apollo, the god of music and medicine, who dictated the laws of choreography, and Terpsichore, daughter of chief-god Zeus and the fifth muse who reigned over the world of dance and choral music.[38] The musings of Greek thinkers, including Pythagoras (c. 570 - c. 495 BC) and Lucian, the second-century Greek writer of Assyrian origins (circa 120 – 200 AD), also fed the notion of a "dancing universe" presided over by terpsichorean deities.[39] Early thinkers such as Thales and Heraclitus postulated early conceptions of a "dancing universe," contending all is in dynamic motion and constant change in a "world of becoming."[40] This approach effectively rejected the errant view held by Parmenides and his fellow Eleatics, who maintained reality was static and immutable. [41] Pythagoras (circa 585 AD -), an amalgam of mathematician, musician, and mystic, divined an ordered and pattern universe from performing the lyre.[42] While Pythagoras and his followers were jamming in the Italian city of Croton, he noted certain combinations of string lengths created beautiful sounds while others did not, and further observed there were common ratios underlying musical harmony.[43] Consequently, Pythagoras postulated a universe consisting of "numbers dancing according to mathematical relationships," the dance of the numbers as it were, that gave the universe a rational explanation.[44] For his part, Lucian wrote that dance played a pivotal role at the creation, linking "the mysteries" at the beginning of the world itself, with the ordered and harmonious movements of the heavens, mirroring the first dance at the genesis.[45] He opined the universe and dance were born together, signaling "the union of the elements," including the beautiful and structured movements of the dance of the stars and the planets.[46] The notion that the stars and planets were engaged in the cosmic dance of the heavens was manifested in the astral dances of ancient Egypt priests - a theme also captured in an astral ballet choreographed by Leonardo Da Vinci.[47] As Marcelo Gleiser observed, the dancing universe of the ancients was not just an allegorical portrayal of the medium and mystery creation; it actually represented a potent animating force that impacted every aspect of life. [48]

In a cosmogony governed by a pantheon of dancing deities, it was natural for humans who received the gift of dance from the gods to pay them homage through ritual dance. As Lucian observed, "what delights the gods must delight man."[49] Since the aboriginal ritual dances initiated by choreographer-gods and goddesses, dance has been a mainstay of human affairs, fulfilling a range of needs, including communicating with the spiritual world, healing rituals, and just plain entertainment. For example, the Greeks honored their deities during rituals such as the famed Dionysian spring festival marked by processions of dancers, singers, officiating priests, and revelers in ceremonies reminiscent of the Egyptians' celebrations in honor of Isis.[50] Incidentally, the modern carnival gets its etymological birth from the Carrus Navalis, the ancient ship on wheels used during a ceremony to recreate the life, death, and return of Dionysius.[51]

*****

At the zenith of ancient Greek civilization, dance was a well-established fixture in all communal activities, including medicine, healing, and health. Dance played a pivotal role in ancient Greece, affecting diverse spheres

of life, including education, arts, politics, philosophy,

health, and physical fitness. Greeks from high society to

lowly places were enamored with dance and eager to

dance at every opportunity. Greek gods danced a storm.

Philosophers rationalized dance in discourse; poets and

singers eulogized dance in moving verses, statesmen

strutted their stuff, and accomplished dancers were the

envy of all.[52]   Lucian, the Greek/Assyrian writer,

opined: "...the most noble and greatest personages in

every city are the dancers, and so little are they

ashamed of it, that they applaud themselves more upon

their dexterity in that species of talent than on their

nobility, their posts of honor, and the dignities of their

forefathers."[53] Statesmen, generals, philosophers,

poets, and other important personages performed solo

dances in front of massive audiences at major public

events. For example, Sophocles, who was renowned for

creating his own original choreography and for solo

dancing proclivities, performed a historic victory dance

at the conclusion of the battle.[54] Similarly, Aeschylus

and Aristophanes danced in performances of their

plays, and Thespis and Euripides were notable

choreographers as well.[55] The central role of dance in

Greek life made ancient Greece civilization the standard

for other societies, the inspirational archetype for

proponents of dance through the ages, and,

concomitantly, the bane for future antagonists of

dance.[56]

With regimens that were very physically demanding,

the Greeks apotheosized the importance of fitness

through dance. As Walter Sorell wrote, "To the Greeks,

dancing was a means of achieving health in every part

of the body; it was a rhythmic ball game…"[57] Greek

philosophers, thinkers, and poets also expounding on

the connections between dance, fitness, and battle readiness for the polis.[58] Plato (427–347 BC) considered physical activities such as dancing and other exercises as sister arts to medicine.[59] Pythagoras (570-495 BC) theorized music could restore proper balance among the four humors in some patients and contribute to a more balanced life with greater bodily and mental health.[60] Hippocrates (460–377 BC) stated that the best way to maintain health is to dedicate the whole day to increasing one's strength through physical exercise.[61] Galen (129–217 AD), the renowned Greek physician, wrote extensively about aerobic fitness associated with Greek acrobatic dances and muscle strength.[62] Moreover, the link between physical fitness, dance, and war-preparedness was a central feature in Greek civilization, with dance prowess directly linked to bravery, martial ability, and victory in battle.[63] For example, the dance of the Curetes vividly illustrated the powerful combination of physical intensity and martial influence that was so emblematic of Greek ritual dances.[64] In some battles, the commander in charge of designing and executing battle strategies was also the dance leader.[65] In the Iliad, Homer describes the seeming invincibility of a brave fighter named Meriones; the Cretan, who danced while engaged in battle, "could not be hit by a lance or stone."[66] Young Spartans from the age of five were required to practice a weapon dance, combining gymnastics, exercise, and instruction in battle strategies. [67]

Leading Greek philosophers opined on dance education and its impact on the development of youth and the health of the polis. Greek dance instruction, which involved vigorous exercise, was deemed a fundamental building block of a healthy and robust society; as Plato put it, "to sing and to dance well is to be well educated."[68] Plato believed "the sense of harmony and rhythm" that creates dance out of "natural and instinctive movements" is a gift of the gods and the Muses that required cultivating and refinement.[69] Furthermore, he maintained all creatures innately used rhythmic movement to express feelings, noting that certain dances ennoble the motions of physically attractive bodies while others parody the motions of "ugly bodies."[70] Plato recommended instruction in "noble dances" that conferred not only "health and ability and beauty of the body, but also goodness of the soul and a well-balanced mind."[71] Likewise, Socrates, who confessed to dancing alone at dawn and wished for greater skill in the "graceful art" of dance, recommended dance be more widely taught.[72] Socrates argued dance was necessary "for health, for complete and harmonious physical development, for beauty, for the ability to give pleasure to others, for reducing the acquisition of good appetite, for the enjoyment of sound sleep."[73] Moreover, Socrates favored dance instruction for future soldiers because he believed the best dancers made the best warriors.[74] Meanwhile, Aristotle supported education in dance after age fourteen because it afforded immense intellectual and aesthetic benefits and helped purge youth's souls of "unseemly emotions." [75] He believed dance more effectively expressed the action in the Greek tragedies as it brought out the pathos and ethos of the characters and prepared the citizen for appropriate enjoyment of leisure.[76] In light of the Greek record on dancing for health and fitness, it is no surprise that the noted physician Hieronymus Mercurialis, author of the first text of modern physical education - De Arte Gymnastica (1569) – called for a revival of the physical education regimen of the Greeks. [77]

*****

While Greek civilization put a high premium on dancing ability, its neighbor and rival, Imperial Rome, looked at the dance with askance, treating it as entirely unbecoming, even an un-Roman, activity that posed a threat to public order.[78] In particular, the Roman upper class had a snobbish and dismissive attitude towards dancing, viewing it as an unsuitable and unproductive activity that was beneath their high status.[79] Expressing the "priggish-puritanical feeling" about dance typical of Imperial Rome's ruling class, Cicero (106-43 B.C.) lambasted the degeneracy of dance, stating "...nobody dances, unless he be drunk or a madman."[80] Referring to an honorable Roman as a dancer was tantamount to slander, and, undoubtedly, an aspersion most vile.[81] Guardians of public morals often sought to ban all dancing because they were concerned it could weaken the mettle of Roman youth and even compromise their training as warriors for the Empire.[82] Whereas leading Greek statesmen, philosophers and poets used dancing ability as an indicia of accomplishment and status, Romans relegated dance to the realm of mere popular entertainment for their slaves, captives, and presumably uncivilized foreigners.[83] Roman ambivalence towards dance gave scandal-mongers a field day when it was discovered that prior to her marriage, Theodora, the notorious wife of emperor Justinian I, had performed naked as a dancer in a circus.[84] Since Byzantine law prohibited patricians from marrying entertainers, Justinian I had to persuade the reigning emperor, Justin, to legally confer patrician status on Theodora, a cover-up involved considerable "legal acrobatics."[85] Incidentally, Nero, who fancied himself a great dancer, and Caligula, both pandered to the Roman public's fascination with mimes, to the consternation of Roman leaders such as Marcus

Aurelius.[86] Dance was viewed more favorably in the Empire between 200-150 BC - a relatively brief period during which Etruscan and Greek choreographers taught Roman patrician children in private schools.[87] Unfortunately, the reprieve was short-lived: Emperor Scipio Aemilianus Africanus closed Roman dance schools around 150 B.C., reacting to fears dance would weaken the mettle of Roman citizens.[88] Thus, unlike the Greeks, official Rome made little contribution to the advancement of dance, save for the refinement of pantomime spectacles, the easily understandable dance-dramas dependent on elaborate movement sequences, and gestures instead of speech.[89] These spectacles were so popular they survived the closure of the dancing schools, albeit degenerating into cheap eroticism towards the end of the Empire.[90]

Although dance lacked the official imprimatur in Rome, the populace found ways to dance, sometimes emulating or creating new versions of Greek dance rituals. Lacking both elite sanction and support, dancing in Imperial Rome was primarily relegated to tawdry spectacles that delivered "brutal and sensationalized" excitement for the general populace.[91] Dance by non-Roman slaves was also a feature in the public games of the Empire, while foreigners often danced in the northern provinces and Sicily.[92] Meanwhile, Roman masses adopted several Greek rituals and festivals, including appropriating Dionysus (renamed Bacchus) along with the panoply of dancing maenads and satyrs for the notorious bacchanalia.[93] Other important Roman dance rituals and festivals included the Salii (holy processions to honor Mars), Lupercalia, Ludiones and Saturnalia.[94] Beginning December 17th and lasting an entire week, Saturnalia, the famous pagan festival, was marked by wild dancing and debauchery to honor

Saturnus, the god of farming and agriculture.[95] The free-

for-all libertinism in the "dance of primal ecstasy"

during Saturnalia was a display of "sexual hedonism"

that also contributed to a new genre of lustful cabarets

for popular entertainment.[96] Charitable giving occurred

during Saturnalia, and distinctions between masters

and bondsmen were blurred as both sat and dined

together, serving each other.[97]

As the Roman Empire collapsed, the emerging Church

had to contend with a web of time-worn ancient dance

rituals for good fortune and health, many of which were

intricately embedded in a web of cultural traditions

going back many centuries.[98] The tableau of offending

ritual dance practices included festivities featuring

Persian divinities as the sun-god Mithra, Cybelic rites,

Druid ceremonies, Teutonic dance rites, astral dances,

serpent-imitating rituals, Dionysian bacchanals, and Saturnalia.[99] Many of these rites had become so popular that they blended seamlessly into the social and cultural landscape, including the popular Maypole dances, Shrovetide, fire dances, ring-dances to greet the sunrise, and fertility rituals where dancers regularly donned charms for good fortune.[100] While expressing its strong disapproval, the Church also became quite adept at finding accommodation with many ancient traditions, effectively winning converts by grafting aspects of old pagan dance rituals to Christian concepts. [101] For example, the Church adroitly co-opted many popular European mid-winter dramatic performances that generally shared common themes involving the struggle between life and death, culminating in revival after death. [102] Teutonic rites of dawn (Eastre) morphed to Easter; the Druids' tree-adoring ceremonies and their burning of yule logs were absorbed into the rites of

Christmas, requiring a "a shift in the date of the birth of Christ."[103] Certain aspects of the Saturnalia festival and its gift exchange practice were later adopted by Christians for Christ's Mass or Christmas.[104]

*****

In a world where music, singing, and dance were central components of rituals, the quest for health, healing, and good fortune generally, was typically a communal event. The infirm were usually situated in the center of a communal ring dance and encircled until dancers in "an ecstatic state" overwhelmed the "spirit of sickness."[105] For example, the famed Navajo dance to cure diseases known as "medicine sings" were elaborate affairs that brought people of the community together.[106] The ceremonies that went on for nine days included prayers and the creation of sand-paintings in secret, sweat baths, and medications for the sick.[107] In India, communities held intricate serpent rituals presided over by a special caste of priests restore health, including warding off blindness, dermatological conditions, or just plain ill-fortune.[108] Among the Gran Chaco people, the infirm person sometimes danced in a circle of community members as part of the healing ritual.[109] In one account, sick Toba women danced "faster and faster" within a circle of singing townspeople, "until the sickness spirits escape[d] in perspiration" and were chased off into the woods by men brandishing firebrands.[110] Among the Ute native people of North America, community members "create[d] healing power against rheumatism" by dancing around a sun pole.[111] In nineteenth-century France, children suffering from hernias in the Seine-et-Oise region were carried under an oak tree where women danced around them in ritual healing ceremonies.[112] Mothers in Barjols (France) participated in a healing dance during Marcellus Day's high mass dance; they lifted their newborn babies and swung them in a circle in an ecstatic frenzy to promote health and growth.[113]

These and other ritual dances helped bond the individual with the community and reflected a powerful expression of social identity, group affinity, kinship, or sense of belonging. As Krauss observed, dance, community, and individual identity were so inextricably bound together that among the Bantu of Africa that instead of asking, "Who are you?" the more relevant question was, "What do you dance?"[114] Anthropologists like Margaret Mead and Alan Merriam marvel at the central importance of dance in ancient civilizations, viewing it as vital to understanding culture.[115] The fellowship of dance was also a celebration of kinship, cementing bonds of group affinity and solidarity that

helped define one's tribe and its distinctiveness from

other tribes. Besides expressing tribal identity and the

sense community, Medearis concluded dance helped

identify the individual's proper role in a group and their

place in the wider community.[116] As Merriam

proclaimed, "dance is culture and culture is dance...The

entirety of dance is not separable from the

anthropological concept of culture."[117] Through

ancestral dances passed down from generation to

generation, humans strengthened communal bonds,

developed "social affirmation," and provided the

community a unifying sense of shared experience.[118]

In this context, researchers suggest ritual dance

emerged through the ages as a primary force for social

organization, with numerous rituals commemorating all

aspects of life, including paying homage to the gods and

celebrations of bountiful harvests, hunts, weddings, births, and funerals.[119] First and foremost, communal ritual dance was the pervasive and predominant mode of spiritual communication with the gods.[120] The dance was the medium that bound people to each other and their gods, ancestors, and community; dancing together in communal rituals was key to a group's overall success.[121] Dance and ritual movement manifested and conveyed "unspoken group values" intrinsic to the tribe's experience, making it unnecessary to articulate them in conventional literal and rectilinear ways.[122] Thus, Jean Laude observed dance initiated the process of clarifying, preserving and transmitting "original knowledge," that German philosophers refer to as Urnatur.[123] In this context, the dance bequeaths the community a "framework of common experience," as well as inter-generational solidarity, connecting past, present, and future.[124] The power of communal ritual dance shaped the community's collective spirit and soul; its character and portrait were etched in choreographic patterns and postures passed down from generation to generation. Through ritual dances, people experienced more than just fellowship and solidarity; they sang and danced together as they celebrated, commiserated, and mourned, commemorating all events in the continuum of the arc of life.[125] In effect, dance connected and even sublimated the individual to the communal, helping to build more cohesive communities where people were not dancing alone in the void. In healing dance ceremonies where people came together to propitiate the gods and importune them for good fortune, dancing was inextricably bound with community fellowship. Moreover, healing dance rituals could not be divorced from their sacred underpinnings; the dance was a medium of communication, not just in the here-and-now but also with the divine realm.[126]

*****

Given the mind-body-spirit nexus in ritual dances, dance historian Walter Sorell contends they cannot be understood without contemplating the religious, spiritual, and otherworldly themes enacted in descriptive gestures and reflective bodily symbols. [127] For example, traditional Hindu-inspired dances involve significant mind-body connection, transforming the body itself into the "embodied soul" that deploys the hands, the voice, and the mind to convey its passions and desires; it appears as if the body is thinking.[128] Elaborate Sanskrit classical dance-dramas rooted in Hindu teachings such as the Bharatanatyam developed around the 5th century AD, established a ritualized mind-body language, including arcane hand movements (mudras) and complex facial expressions to tell stories of relations with the gods.[129] Steeped in recherché aesthetics, the Bharatanatyam is renowned for meticulously expressive gestures assigned to various body parts representing specific themes and emotions.[130] There are an astounding twenty movements allotted to the head alone, four to the neck and six to eyebrows and twenty-four to the eyes, and fifty-seven hand movements related to various dance contexts in prescriptive ways.[131] The dance, which is mostly performed by females, requires extensive training. [132] Meanwhile, the Kathakali - a dance drama and Hindu passion play - was first performed by Brahmin priests, who illustrated the legends of their faith with dramatic pantomimic presentations.[133] Mostly performed on the west coast of South India, the Kathakali is often staged by men and boys (playing female roles). [134] Performers don elaborate costumes and use hand gestures and spoken words to recount tales of deities, demons, and heroes from the two great Hindu epics, the Ramayana and Mahabharata. [135] These dances have spread across the subcontinent to places like Cambodia, where performers engage in convulsive dances with fluid marionette-like movements and body distortions while displaying similarly intricate hand gestures and sublime expressions.[136]

Some ritual dances of possession, where the dancer seeks to be possessed by a spirit, serve as a medium of communication with otherworldly forces and for healing, release, and transcendence from earthly torments.[137] During the crescendo of sacred dances, a participant may be overcome and even transformed into a spirit or ancestral deity, making the dancer an avatar of the god as well as an instrumentality for the deity's message, predilection, or revelation.[138] In these trance-like ritual dances of possession, the border between mind-body-spirit is blurred as dancers are moved to ecstatic transcendence by the overpowering spiritual force. [139] This "genuine" possession that effectively bridges the nature-culture "antithesis" is usually an intense, physical, and overwhelming phenomenon, with the possessed fainting or mimicking the symptoms of epilepsy and displaying melodramatic fervor.[140] Among the Yoruba Orisha cult (as well as the Haitian voodoo or the Brazilian Candomble societies), dance rituals peak at the height of possession where a participant may be transformed into the horse of the genie, spirit, or deity.[141] In the process, the dancer who experiences hysteria becomes unconscious and subsequently "opens himself to the spirit," performing repetitive dance moves that cause him to be directed by the spirit and simulate its unique physical traits.[142] Although ritual dancers did not often know whether, by whom, or what form the possession would take, they

readied themselves to execute the entirety of steps

directed by the possessing deity or ancestor who chose

to control or ride them. [143]   Being possessed by a deity

or ancestor during ritual dance was such a great honor

that among certain tribal peoples, it was a precondition

for participation in the dances of secret societies.[144]

Some ecstatic ritual dances veered on the impossible.

In the state of possession, elements of mysticism, magic,

and hypnosis combine, enabling dancers to overcome

fear and achieve superhuman feats as they transcended

their bodies.[145] For example, possessed dancers in

Sudan formed a dance circle and "swallow[ed] burning

coals;" Sri Lankan fire dancers blanketed themselves in

flames "without being burned," and other held flaming

torches down their throats.[146] Similarly, the Luiseno

Native American Indians of California walked barefoot

on glowing embers with impunity.[147] Voodoo dancers in the West Indies pressed their bare skin on glowing irons, remaining unaffected.[148] Trance dancers of Indonesia thrust sharp daggers against their bare breasts without injury.[149] Elsewhere, wrench dances common among the Siberian Ostyak and West African Fan peoples involved a superhuman distortion of the body, including contorted movements so out of harmony with the norm that the dancer effectively became "a puppet on strings."[150] Among the ritual dances that continue to astound viewers to this day are the stupendous whirling dances of the Sufis, who perform a sublime reality-transcending to experience oneness with God and total happiness by spinning non-stop for up to fifteen hours.[151]

Equally impressive are the intrepid ritual leap dances for health and good fortune, acrobatic feats that appear to defy gravity. For example, Africa, that Curt Sachs dubbed "the continent of the leap dance," people performed expansive skyward leaps akin to the towering spires of great Gothic Cathedrals like Notre Dame.[152] In this context, the leaps symbolize a yearning for escape from the torments of this world, effectively kinetic entreaties for a deus ex machina in the struggle against the albatross of the human condition.[153] Common among many African peoples, including the Yoruba of Nigeria, leap dances were believed to promote health, crop growth, fertility, and life renewal.[154] Similarly, various tribes in Africa, ancient Mexico, and the Kurnai people of S.E. Australia engaged in ritualistic lift dances where children were hoisted high up in the air to appeal to the gods to make the children grow taller, stronger, and healthier.[155]

Even with advances in modern science and technology, ritual healing dance traditions continue to flourish in many parts of the world. For example, across parts of Africa, ritual healing dances still play a crucial role as a therapeutic outlet as they have done for millennia. [156] In an article published in the Journal of Panafrican Studies in 2011, Nicole Monteiro and her colleagues demonstrated that these medicinal dances are intense communal affairs that bridge the gap between the material and spiritual, with dancing itself serving as the portal to the realm of supernatural forces underlying all phenomena.[157] Medicine men and shamans on the fringes of modernity are still presumed to possess supernatural powers to connect with the netherworld's ancestral spirits, seek favor from the gods, ward off illnesses, cure diseases, and cast off bad omens and bring solace to the infirm. [158] To better understand contemporary African ritual healing dances, Monteiro and her team examined the Ndeup ritual in Senegal, the

Zar tradition in Northeast Africa, and the highly stylized

dance techniques of Guinea. [159] The researchers

explored the role of these dances in coping with trauma,

focusing particularly on how ritual dance ceremonies

"integrate social, spiritual, physical, and mental realms."

[160] The researchers found that ritual dances reduced

trauma by heightening intersubjective empathy, causing

dancers to shift emotional states as rapid dance

movements helped induce detached states of

consciousness and cathartic release.[161] For example,

the Senegalese Ndeup is a healing ritual for villagers

possessed by spirits to reconcile with the ancestors,

purify or cleanse themselves and obtain protective

shields against evil spirits. [162] The Zar healing

ceremony in Northeast Africa relies on dancing, singing,

drumming, and induction of trance-like states to help

persons who are possessed by the Zar spirit. [163] Once a

Zar possession or affliction is diagnosed, the afflicted person who cannot shake off the life-long association with his/her particular Zar spirit is required and expected to engage in the annual ceremony to propitiate the Zar spirit. [164] In communal dance rituals lasting hours or even days, ritual offerings are presented to appease the spirits and lessen the trauma of affliction and actual possession by the Zar.[165]

In these contexts, ritual dance provides a high-speed connection to the gods, linking human supplicants to their ancestors and deities of the nether world. For example, during the Egungun ritual, where the Yorubas of Benin commemorate the Return of the Spirit of Death, participants believe their dances opened direct lines of communication to their ancestral spirits.[166] The Egungun, who belong to both the world of the living and the dead, were spirits of deceased kings and heads of

families who descended to earth to help humans.[167]
During the ceremony, the spirits are portrayed by men
wearing long garb and ceremonial headgear while
spinning and stamping feet, in a manner reminiscent of
their personalities when they were alive.[168] Their
elaborate costumes are festooned with magnificent long
stoles and cloth strips that seem to come to life in
auspicious winds that bring "security and the promise
of fortune."[169]   Similarly, the nexus between the present
and the spirit world is reinforced in the ritual
celebration of the Guere of the Ivory Coast's Guiglo
region, where participants dance to restore order and
calm to a chaotic world.[170] During the ceremony,
participants celebrate the revered Gbona gla, the "great
mask of wisdom," traceable to a ritual dance at the
creation when man sought relief from the constant
strife that impeded efforts to build a stable and well-
ordered society.[171]   In response, the god of creation,

Nyon sua, sent forth good spirits to earth, which provided humans the ability to live a well-ordered, prosperous and healthy life by laying down society's laws; these laws were subsequently revealed in the mask of wisdom.[172] Therefore, any time society falls prey to distress, akin to the torments at the dawn of creation, the Guere invoke the masks at the origin of the world. Given the mask's association with the gods, they can reconcile feuding parties, control witches, ward off illnesses, cast off evil spirits, and re-assert order.[173]

Ancient ritual dances appeared to blur any distinction between the physical material realm and the spiritual sphere. Consider, for example, the dance for health and good fortune by the followers of Osun, the Yoruba river goddess. [174] The dancers participate in a ritual procession to a river to offer Osun her favorite foods and spices and importune her to cure ailments and ensure fertility.[175] In this context, our contemporary "dualist" framework that draws a bright line between "secular and religious, profane and sacred" makes it difficult to comprehend ancient ritual dances and their significance fully.[176] Participants of ritual dances largely shared a "pantheistic and animistic belief in a world of essences which is embodied in all forces and elements," a "fundamental power," aka nature, or what the Iroquois called orenda, the "supernatural energy inherent in everything in the world."[177] In this context, Jamake Highwater contends the dancing body amplifies its senses in a physiological "process of perception and thought by which brain recreates itself as mind," effectively transforming the body into a spirited being inherently capable of spiritual engagement in a spirited world.[178] Thus, Huett observed that in ritual dances where "art is indistinguishable from life," dance exemplifies the profound "communion between man and the universe."[179] Occupying a realm outside the boundaries of civilization, ritual dance in ancient societies belonged to a mysterious other sphere or "second world."[180] This sphere is effectively a coterminous, overlapping, parallel dimension that is a sacred fount of ritual knowledge the gateway to "many separate realities" of a "multi-verse, or a bi-verse but not the traditional uni-verse of Western civilization."[181] In these ancient dance cultures, the celebration of the physical body was also unmoored from approaches that viewed the body as the fount of sin, freeing it to explore the fullness of consciousness without boundaries. As Jamake Highwater described it, for many of these cultures, mind/spirit and body/flesh are united in harmony with nature and fully integrated into a world where everything is alive. The ancient dancers like the Greeks who "idealized man" celebrated the body and believed it was endowed with high-minded qualities, including aspirational thinking, genuine feelings, and ideals.[182] In this context, the dancing body's expressive force is at once sacred and mysterious because "ideas and feelings are merged in the spiritual body."[183] The primitive dancer, perhaps donning an animal mask was completely transported to an ecstatic dimension where dancing constitutes spontaneous and religious self-expression that is fully integrated into his/her life.[184] Such was the case in the secret dance rituals of the Bambara tribesmen of Mali who donned animal masks, or various 'medicine man' healing dances as well as ritual tree-worshipping dances to propitiate deities; dancing was the thing itself.[185] As the foregoing suggests, the practice of ritual dance medicine goes beyond physical movement, bringing together mind, body, and spirit. As the preceding suggests, keener insights into the intricate mind-body-spirit alignment at the heart of the dance could maximize the psychological, emotional, and social benefits of dance.

Recall that neuroscientist Ivar Hagendoorn declared

that while the limbs move, "it is the brain that

dances."[186] True. But, besides the limbs and the brain,

and, the spirit or the soul also dances. As L.S.

Ramaswamy Sastri stated, dance is "not mere activity of

the human limbs...It is the embodied soul's attempt to

express not only through the mind and the senses alone

... but through the mind and senses and body acting

together, its nature and its visions."[187]

Through ritual dance, people paid tribute to the divine

in their temples, churches, and shrines where they

moved, processed, circled, and leaped in ecstasy before

their deity. The dance as a sacred art was guided by

priests, shamans, holy men, and women, from ziggurats

of the ancient Sumerians to the temples of the ancient

Egyptians and Greeks to contemporary Whirling

Dervishes. The Old Testament and the Talmud describe many "ritual processions, whirling, hooping dances, harvest dances, and wedding dances" – although men and women danced separately.[188] Biblical Hebrew contains at least a dozen verbs to describe dancing, although the most frequently used was "hul" or "hil" meaning "to whirl" or to turn; the Hebrew word for festival, "hagag," also translates to "to move in a circle," suggesting a circle dance.[189] At any rate, biblical peoples were enamored with ritual dance celebrations and received some very authoritative exhortations.[190] In the book of Exodus, Jewish prophets celebrated their relationship with God by dancing, using symbolic movement as an effective tool in communicating the divine message.[191] The Bible also contains a prophecy as enunciated by Rabbi Elazar, to wit, "Someday the Holy One ...will give a dance for the righteous..."[192] For example, Isaiah 55:12 clearly urges the faithful to celebrate in song and dance: "You shall go out with joy and be led forth in peace: The mountains and the hills shall break forth into singing, and all trees of the field clap their hands."[193] Memorable dance occasions include the wedding "dance of the Mahanaim," (Song of Solomon 6:13) and the daughters of Shiloh coming out to "dance in dances" at the annual vintage festival (Judges 12:21). To celebrate King Herod's birthday, Salome "danced before him and his guests and pleased Herod." as noted in Mathew 14:6.[194] Meanwhile, Miriam and other women celebrated after crossing the Red Sea as Miriam grabbed a timbrel, followed by all the women each "with timbrels and with dances." In Psalms 149:3, people are urged to dance: "Let them praise His name in the dance: let them sing praises unto Him with timbrel and harp."[195] Elsewhere, Jeremiah 31:13 states, "Then shall the virgin rejoice in the dance, both young men and old together: for I will turn their mourning into joy, and will comfort them, and make them rejoice from their sorrow." To top it all, to celebrate the Ark, King David only partially clothed "with a linen ephod," danced before the Lord in "a rotary dance" as part of a "religious procession, organized in honor of Jahwe." The great King performed for the Lord with all his might, skipping with joy, "leaping and dancing," unquestionably an ecstatic "skip dance," "accentuated by violent leaps" of joy.[196] (6 Samuel 14 -21; 1 Chronicle 15:29) In his classic text, The Dance Through the Ages, Walter Sorell draws a striking parallel between King David's attire while dancing before the Ark to the Prophet Mohammad who was "clothed with no more than the ihram'" as he moved in a circle with other pilgrims around the Kaaba.[197] Dr. Omid Safi, the eminent scholar and director of Duke University's Islamic Studies Center, has also described the circumambulation of the Kaaba itself as, in part, a "dance," noting stating, "A beautiful circle is formed, moving round and round in adoration of God. It is a walk, a dance, a prayer rolled into one… the whole rest of the world is caught up in an ecstatic whirling. Here is the stillness, the axis of the world, around which all dance, activity, motion takes place."[198]

Various historical accounts of gnostic gospels and hymns including the Acts of St. John alluded to a dancing deity.[199] In gnostic gospels, Jesus enjoined his disciples to dance as part of worship, effectively elevating dance to the level of prayer for the blessings of life and salvation. In one passage, he proclaimed, "Grace danceth. I would pipe; dance ye all…The Whole on high hath part in our dancing. Amen. Whoso danceth not, knoweth not what cometh to pass. Amen…Now answer thou unto my dancing…Thou that dancest, perceive what I do …"[200] This dancing Jesus exhorts the faithful to dance, proclaiming, "If you cannot equate yourself with God, You cannot know him, for like is known by like."[201] Furthermore, in Luke 6:23, Jesus in the New Testament endorses joyous and expressive movements akin to dance, telling his followers "to rejoice and leap for joy" in celebration of the return of the prodigal son.[202] According to linguistic experts, the words 'rejoice' and 'dance' were used interchangeably in Aramaic.[203] Elsewhere Luke 7:32, states, "We have piped unto you, and ye have not danced..." – a statement that inspired Ambrose, Bishop of Milan in the 4th century, who "wrote profusely in support of church dance."[204] Eusebius, the father of church history also wrote about sacred dancing in the early (pre-Constantine) Church. [205] Describing the worship of the Therapeuts by Philo, he wrote: "...they chant hymns composed in God's honor...now dancing to the measure and now inspiring it, at times dancing in procession, at times set-dances, and then circle dances right and left."[206] Nonetheless, as the early Church moved determinedly against the pagan ways of Graeco-Roman life, it propounded the new Christian theology that considered the human body a vessel of sin, and that prioritized the spirit over the flesh.[207] Consequently, the Church opposed pagan rituals like dance, deeming it an evil to be condemned or banned in various edicts, including at the Council of Toledo in 539 A.D and other subsequent councils.[208]

*****

Two thousand years after Greek ruminations about dancing deities in a dancing universe, Albert Einstein picked up the thread with profound insights about the dance. Designating dancers as "the athletes of God," he declared that all things in the universe, including cosmic dust, are "dancers" in an enigmatic choreographic performance.[209] Einstein's pronouncements about dance reinforce the underlying spiritual or sacred dimension of dance energy, virtually elevating it into a fifth fundamental force of sorts. As Einstein proclaimed, "we all dance to a mysterious tune, intoned in the distance by an invisible piper."[210] In that regard, the appreciating and mirroring the movement of which are part of is the least we can do as the athletes of the cosmic force that is expressed through constant motion. We are all dancers in this cosmogony, dancers in a dancing universe. At the initial dance of quantum soup, the primal kinetic act of creation, the Invisible Piper's rhythmic riffs triggered quantum fluctuations, string vibrations, and ripples pregnant with infinite energy. The original dance of coquetry between matter and anti-matter took place on a pebble-sized discotheque that contained and constituted everything. Egged on by the Einstein's "Invisible Piper," aka DJ Moving-Mover, all particles foamed and frothed, whipping themselves into a frenzied dance that culminated in the most incredible light show that ever was, the evidence of it still lodged in the cosmic microwave background. The cognoscenti have since called that august shindig the Big Bang, but whatever you might want to call it, it certainly was magnificent shebang! It has been nearly 14 billion years since, but that dance goes on, and we are still in it. Since that grand debut, we have been part and parcel of the cosmic ball, atoms, molecules, particles, waves, wave-like particles, and particles cross-dressing as waves - prancing, pirouetting, and parading on the fabric of time and space. Behold the perfect synchronicity of the dance of electrons that quantum entangle each other, suspended in superposition, spinning, and counter-spinning, shuffling and counter-shuffling; leading and following, in perfect unison across the infiniteness of the ether. Light waves illuminate this cosmic dance floor as they lead our awe-inspiring dance across space-time at a mind-warping 186,000 miles per second (670 million miles an hour). Not to be outdone, identical matter and antimatter neutrinos dance their way through everything and nothing, traveling near the speed of light, nary stopping nor interacting for a nanosecond in their carefree dance through the expanding universe. The planet's daily ring dance on its axis reaches speeds up to a thousand miles an hour, and its rotary whirl around our local disco ball occurs at a vertiginous 66,000 miles an hour. Our sun, solar system in tow, is likewise engaged in a fiery round dance around the center of the Milky Way at an astounding 500,000 to 600,000 miles an hour, a feat requiring a staggering 225 million years to complete.[211] The Milky Way itself, spiral arms akimbo, is twirling at 1.4 million miles an hour around the maypole of the universe, towards its fateful tango with Andromeda, or not, depending on the fancy footwork of the Large Magellanic Cloud.[212] As for our funky universe, it continues its all-encompassing dance of inflation. Starlets dance their way to superstardom and go supernovae; galaxies form, hook up, collide and collapse into black holes, triggering gravitational waves that dance across and stretch the very fabric of time and space. Against this backdrop, Albert Einstein's Delphic proclamation is also an exhortation of sorts for us all, dancers, "the athletes of God," to engage in the dance of the universe or the universal spirit. As Aldous Huxley concluded, movement is so completely enmeshed into the nature of things that it is through their muscles that people can "most easily obtain knowledge of the divine."[213]   You do not have to look very far to experience this dancing universe, what with the mosh-pit streaming with energy all around the biome, including molecules that danced off other dancers through the eons. No wonder Cynthia Winton-Henry wrote, "the dancing universe is literally in us;" the entire vastness and motion of the universe are contained in each of us, along with endless spirals of DNA that are worlds onto themselves, "spiral-dancing inside our bodies."[214]

While contemporary dance has lost much of its ritual and sacred underpinnings, understanding the roots of ritual dance through the ages informs appreciation of how dance shaped our evolutionary lineage over tens of thousands of years. Moreover, variants of ancient ritual healing ceremonies still occur in parts of the world, providing participants relief for sundry ailments alternative or complementary therapies. For example, Shiva temples in India also see more people for various ailments alongside modern doctors.[215] Similarly, as Nicole Monteiro and her colleagues showed, ritual medicine dances are still prevalent in parts of Africa.[216] Among the ritual dances that continue to astound viewers to this day are the stupendous and mesmerizing whirling dances of the Sufi Whirling Dervishes or semazens, who perform a sublime reality-transcending to experience oneness with their God, spinning non-stop for hours.[217] The Sufis are followers of Jelaluddin Mohammad Rumi, the 13th-century Persian spiritual leader, and poet, who stated: "Oh Sun God that the master has created, The fiery soul which planets whirl around…. Whoever knoweth the power of the dance, dwelleth in God."[218] Adherents of the religious sect believe by turning counter-clockwise for prolonged periods in a meditative movement that includes a prayer (dhikr or remembrance of God), they will lose themselves as they attain a higher spiritual plane and directly experience God's presence.[219] These stunning kinetic displays of devotion, perhaps more than any other contemporary dance activity, reify the potency of ritual dance movement and its association with the spiritual realm. In this context, dance appears to bridge the worlds of the body and the spirit, with the ritual of dancing central to understanding and participating in the divine's blessings.

V. Dance & Movement Therapy for Alzheimer's, Dementia & Parkinson's

In the absence of cures for dementia, Alzheimer's and Parkinson's, dance, movement and music therapy could be viable complementary or alternative non-pharmacological options for care. While movement, exercise, and dance are by no means cures for these cruel diseases, there is significant evidence that such physical activity can help alleviate suffering and improve quality of life in some cases. To be sure, for those suffering from these diseases and their caregivers who bear enormous, even unsustainable burdens, this is not enough. To achieve needed breakthroughs, we will also need massive funding increases for research institutions and the national will to mount a monumental Manhattan Project-style moonshot initiative. Furthermore, legislators and policymakers must take concrete and consequential steps to deal with the long-term care crisis, including enacting policies and instituting programs to support families and caretakers. In the absence of a cure for dementia, Alzheimer's, and Parkinson's, there is an urgent need for alternative and complementary therapies to support patients, improve quality of life, and increase satisfaction. As the previous chapter showed, dance and music rituals were an intrinsic part of healing ceremonies for millennia. Yet, as the new science of western medicine gained ascendency, the union of medicine and the healing arts was "gradually broken when the art of medicine gave way to the science of medicine."[1] Nonetheless, to the extent that modern dance and movement therapy (DMT) incorporates certain elements of the traditional healing arts, the creative blends of old and new could also yield even better alternative and complementary treatments.

The foundations of Dance and Movement Therapy (DMT) can be traced to the groundbreaking work of Marian Chace, who started a program in the 1940s to help emotionally distressed veterans use dance to express themselves freely.[2] Chace became the first federal dance therapist at St Elizabeth's Hospital, where she used rhythmic movement to help withdrawn and emotionally distressed patients including schizophrenics, aggressive adults, and anti-social individuals suffering from social isolation and disconnectedness.[3] A former Denishawn dancer, she believed dance therapy was the optimal means of helping patients who could not find their voice express themselves through movement.[4] Beginning with a few referrals, she used dance to help her patients strengthen their connection to their own bodies as a critical step towards connecting with the world and finding harmony with others.[5] Chace's successful interventions increased her visibility such that by the early 50s, she had attracted a cadre of dance therapy interns and followers who became the seeds of a rapidly growing movement.[6] In one of the earliest examples of a therapeutic dance academy, Milton Feher, a Broadway performer who studied with Martha Graham, founded the Feher School of Dance and Relaxation in New York City in 1945.[7] Feher's approach emphasized the therapeutic benefits of dance, including relaxation, meditation, posture, body awareness, mind-body harmony and walking correctly in sync with the body's natural motion.[8] Working well into his eighties, Feher transformed many of his patients' lives, enabling them to overcome myriad physical and mental ailments.[9] One of his star students, Ms. Clare Willis, a regular attendee at the Feher School, who kept on dancing until she was over 100 years old, declared: "You can dance every motion in your life... Every motion you do, you can turn into a dance..."[10] Hear! Hear!

In 1966 Marian Chace and her dedicated troupe of fellow practitioners launched the American Dance Therapy Association (ADTA) to support the growing profession of dance/movement therapy.[11] With several thousand members located in all 50 states and worldwide, the ADTA advocates for the development and expansion of DMT training and services, and promotes professional development opportunities and communication among DMTs.[12] The organization also ensures the highest standards of educational, ethical, and credentialing for DMT, advocates for the inclusion of DMT in healthcare, legislative, academic, and research initiatives and has led efforts to have dance therapy recognized as an eligible service under government health programs.[13] The ADTA also works with colleges, universities, and healthcare institutions to increase educational programs for dance therapy, including Dance Therapist Registered (DTR) licenses. [14] Since its founding, DMTs have continued to build on the pioneering work of Marian Chace, using dance as a powerful medium for self-discovery and healing that also opens the door to mutual awareness, empathetic understanding, and a more wholesome engagement with others.[15] Today, DMTs find employment in hospitals, nursing homes, psychiatric institutions, clinics and community health centers working with people afflicted with diseases such as dementia, Parkinson's, and depression.[16]

The American Dance Therapy Association defines dance therapy as the "psychotherapeutic use of movement to promote emotional, social, cognitive and physical integration of the individual."[17] Underlying dance and movement therapy is the notion of cognitive-behavioral interdependence; mind and body are engaged in reciprocal exchange or interaction such that changes in movement affect total functioning.[18] Myrna Washington observed DMT is grounded in the "biopsychosocial model of psychology in which psychological, physiological, and psychosocial domains interact bi-directionally in interdependent and interconnected relationships."[19] The DMT approach builds on neuroscience developments that suggest physical and psychic processes are more interlinked than previously thought and leverages new insights about kinesthetic intelligence, emotional intelligence, and other ways of knowing.[20] Also, DMT embraces embodiment theory that "predicts afferent feedback from movement to affect cognition and behavior," and further recognizes that even supposedly disembodied mental processes are actually physical phenomena.[21] It is thought that emotions are linked to understanding and interpreting physiological or physical sensations and responses, and sensory experiences and motor skills also impact cognitive processes.[22] As every parent knows, children can express themselves through movement long before they can verbalize their experiences. Jean Seibel, a professor of dance therapy, contends since the early experiences and sensations of being held and carried are "encoded in the body," rhythmic movements later in life "can arouse feelings that resonate with these early experiences and bring hidden conflicts into conscious awareness."[23] Since participation in dance and movement impacts overall cognitive and neurobiological functioning, the DMT can help individuals increase sensory awareness of feelings, self-confidence, and self-identity.[24] In the process, the DMT practitioner can help clients rekindle less-used parts of the body and perhaps even redirect such areas to make them more in sync and fully aligned with the whole.[25]

The DMT approach also assumes movement reflects developmental processes as well as patterns of relating to others, giving rise to a focused analysis of movement, whether perceived as expressive, communicative, or adaptive. In effect, DMT explores various forms of "movement behaviour," as revealed in the therapeutic context, and develops appropriate assessments and interventions. For example, practitioners can employ sophisticated analytical tools such as the Kestenberg Movement Profile (KMP) to identify "psychological, developmental, emotional, cognitive and global health/imbalance through movement, observation, notation and interpretation."[26] After an inventory of the individual's movements, the DMT can develop insightful assessments and formulate helpful intervention modalities.[27] Given the nexus between movement and emotion, Payne posits DMT capitalizes on expressive dance as "a medium for growth and integration," such that through dance, "individual worlds become tangible, personal symbolisms are shared, and relationships become visible."[28] Since cultural and personality differences are also reflected in movement, dance provides a great pathway to better perceive individual states as well as the positions, dispositions, and cultural perspectives of others.[29] Thus, dancing can help build capacity for a genuine "kinesthetic experience," including the ability to "imitate, learn, and feel with others," effectively opening up new neural pathways for mutual empathy and solidarity.[30]

The DMT approach further assumes that new and different ways of moving can generate new experiences of being in the world. In effect, developing or gaining new approaches to movement can lead to the acquisition of novel outlooks, sensibilities, and insights into "a preferred way of being." [31] Since movement is a primary impulse that connects to myriad spheres of human development, dance therapists go beyond the mind and the intellect and focus on observing the movements of the body itself and describing most interactions in terms of movement and spatial relations. [32] Thus, according to Young, DMT emerges out of the "ability to kinaesthetically attune and respond to the implicit and explicit movements of another informed by knowledge of one's own body sensations and movements as well as continual observation and assessment of the client's movement."[33] When working with clients, DMT professionals observe and assess a wide range of techniques. They include movement, improvisation, group movement dynamics, rhythmic movement in sync, games, relaxation, non-verbal expression, touch as well as core dance elements of force, flow, time, and space.[34] As ADTA founding member Blanche Evan put it, dance therapy's objective is "the integration of dance with therapy, so that it becomes one."[35] Rather than focus on technique or aesthetics, dance therapy is primarily concerned with the impact of movement on the performer, specifically how a person's unique movements, reflect any conflicts and helps resolve or contain them.[36] Thus, Jennifer Knapp, a clinical counselor and dance movement therapist in Ohio, does not expect or require her clients to have dance skills, but she encourages "communication" with the body, emphasizing the importance of "just being able to move in general, anything to get [the] body moving instead of staying still."[37] The dance therapist is primarily focused on helping the patient use movement to explore, understand, and reveal feelings as well as to find different ways of being and connecting with oneself and the world.[38] When a patient's movements convey passivity and disconnectedness, dance and movement therapy can make a difference: using movement dynamics, the DMT can enable the patient to experience more confidence, centeredness, and assertiveness.[39] Dance therapists tailor their methods to the individual's needs and predilections: some move together with patients in supportive and mirroring roles, while others are empathetic observers. Meanwhile, others engage in their own dancing to reflect what they perceive or facilitate movement by a person or group that is not very comfortable with dancing.[40] The key, as always, is to help the patient express themselves through movement, even if that takes a little creativity and imagination. To enable her shy clients to perform with more confidence, Katrina Semple of New South Wales turned out the lights and encouraged them to try dancing in the dark - as if no one was observing.[41] As Zoe Christian, a dance therapist in Singapore, put it, the realm of dance is "a safe area" away from the strictures of "mainstream society" for people to vent without using words "to express pain, anger, hate and other emotions."[42]

Incorporating diverse epistemological perspectives, contemporary dance, and movement therapy challenge certain assumptions in the Western intellectual tradition.[43] As Nadja Alexander and Michelle LeBaron contend, the DMT approach is effectively a critique of the disembodied 'self,' central to the Cartesian tradition that separates rational/cognitive intelligence from emotional intelligence, and that also rejects "ways of being and knowing that explicitly engage the body."[44] Contemporary neuroscientists view the Cartesian mind-body dichotomy as unsound and recognize that effective thinking and decision-making require an interplay of multiple intelligences.[45] By integrating the mind, the body, and the environment, dance and movement therapy transform the body into a locus and producer of knowledge.[46] In the words of Rainbow Ho-Tin-hung, Hong Kong's first registered dance therapist and a practitioner of "soul dance," the body is like a "library" that can "store our feelings, emotions, and beliefs."[47] The inextricable link between the "know-why" and the "know-how" as situated in "bodily experience and somatic memory" has significant implications for emotional intelligence and movement studies.[48] Firmly grounded in humanism, DMT also has strong underpinnings in a theoretical framework that draws from diverse sources, including Freud, Darwin, Wilhelm Reich, R.L. Birdwhistell, and Rudolf von Laban.[49] Arguably, Laban remains one of the most influential dance movement theorists today, having developed an elaborate theory about the nature and purpose of dance in an orderly world. He coined the term "choreosophy" or wisdom of dance to describe his philosophy of an abstract choreography that captures the dynamism of human nature.[50] In this cosmogony, the dancing body is "organic nature" that "generates dynamic forms that like natural images, can grow, change shape, gain strength, consume each other, fight, split up, or re-form finally achieving order."[51] Laban, who was imbued with "mountain-moving faith in the power of dance," sought to bring order and harmony to the world through dance.[52] Laban believed that in an ideal world, people who attain the state of "needlessness" can enjoy a happy life through "communal thinking, feeling" and participation in "festive exaltation" through dance.[53]

Dance and movement therapy also embrace a holistic social model of health as practitioners focus broadly on the whole person and all dimensions of health, rather than just the disease. [54] It is assumed health is inextricably tied to the way we connect with our world, making society, culture, economics, and environment, including the quality and depth of our social connections, primary determinants of health and well-being. [55] Under this view, the arts are far from a distraction. Rather, Mike White, a fellow in the Centre for Medical Humanities at Durham University, contends the arts can help patients appreciate the challenges they face, enabling them to explore and develop more robust social connections.[56] According to Tom Madden, director of the drama therapy at NUI Maynooth, the "creative therapies" or the "medical humanities," involving the therapeutic application of art as part of patient care, make it possible to "engage clients in psychological, emotional and social change."[57] This approach gives "equal validity to both body and mind," and enables patients to "explore painful and difficult life experiences through an indirect approach and without chemical application."[58] As Bonny Bainbridge Cohen, artist, researcher, and developer of the Body-Mind Centering (BMC) approach to movement, the body, and consciousness stated: "Art in its finest moment is healing, and healing in its finest moment is art." [59]

Early opponents of dance therapy bemoaned the paucity of evidence-based research that showed the efficacy of dance therapy and called for more systematic studies that compared traditional therapy with and without dance therapy.[60] In addition to insufficient evidence, there was general ignorance about the nature of DMT, including the fear that patients would suffer severe injuries from dancing.[61] Outside the United States, there was even greater suspicion of American-style dance therapy during the mid-nineties in countries like Russia and China, where American practitioners encountered significant scientific skepticism as well as several cultural barriers and unusual pedagogical difficulties.[62]   Believing freedom of expression and improvisation are critical to dance therapy, the Americans encouraged their students to engage in freestyle dancing with unstructured movements that freely expressed their innermost feelings – only to discover this approach seemed "totally foreign" to their Russian students. [63] When Russian students were told to "improvise," they reportedly responded by asking, "What do you mean?" [64] As one Russian colleague, Irina Frulova, put it: "It's not in our culture to listen to our body. There's no room to feel. We are always thinking, thinking, thinking and blocking out any feelings that might get in the way." [65] Reflecting on the challenges, Irina Zinchenko, Russia's top psychiatrist at the time, dismissed dance therapy's claims as "totally unproven" while also lamenting she lacked the funding and personnel needed to undertake a systematic review of the claims.[66] Meanwhile, American-style DMT was also met with a great deal of skepticism in China's professional psychiatric community where concerns were expressed about the suitability of western-style DMT.[67] One Chinese psychiatrist cautioned that DMT might not be well suited for people unaccustomed to "revealing themselves in front of others, let alone dancing around to express themselves."[68] In retrospect, initiatives to introduce western-style dance therapy could have done a better job of recognizing, embracing, and integrating China's rich heritage of healing arts. After all, the Chinese character for medicine contains the one for music, symbolizing the historical link.[69]

*****

After facing much skepticism for much of its history, dance therapy is today a more acceptable adjunct to psychotherapy across many parts of the world. The U.S.

government has even supported the use of dance

therapy in several rehabilitative programs for

veterans.[70] Symbolizing the changing environment,

several healthcare organizations have formed

innovative interdisciplinary partnerships with the arts

featuring dancers, musicians, choreographers, and

neurosurgeons working together to improve patient

care.[71] For example, in Ontario Province, Canada, dance

therapists work with other artists, comics, and

musicians to incorporate the healing arts into the

University Health Network's Open Lab center.[72] Today,

dance and movement therapists are increasingly

involved in non-pharmacological interventions for

managing patient care for patients with Alzheimer's,

dementia, and Parkinson's Disease. Recent research

breakthroughs in dance science, particularly new

insights about how dance affects the brain, have

contributed to greater recognition, and, quite frankly,

greater respect, for DMT. In the absence of cures for Alzheimer's and dementia, it is necessary to explore alternative and complementary non-pharmacological options for improving patient care and well-being, including music and dance therapy. As demonstrated above, there is compelling evidence showing that movement and dance are neurologically impactful and can contribute to positive health outcomes, especially in treating dementia, Alzheimer's, and Parkinson's. Dance therapy is gaining greater legitimacy as an alternative treatment because of the increase in evidence-based research and the testimonials of lived experiences of patients whose lives have been positively affected by movement, exercise, and dance.[73] It is becoming more apparent that dance and movement therapy could be a viable alternative or complementary therapies for wide-ranging ailments, including care for dementia, Alzheimer's, and Parkinson's. In addition to the medicinal impact of the movement itself, dance therapy is particularly well-suited to helping people with neurodegenerative disorders who often have difficulties communicating their innermost thoughts and feelings.[74] In addition to helping patients use movement as medicine for the underlying disease, DMTs can also help patients confront the depression that oft attends chronic diseases, sometimes even getting withdrawn and sedentary patients to re-engage with the world.[75] By enabling patients to express their feelings using movement, they can more readily unearth latent emotions and open pathways to profound personal insights that serve as a basis for further exploration in traditional therapy.[76] Thus, DMTs "working on a body level" can be helpful with certain patients when conventional approaches have not succeeded, occasionally obtaining significant results such as getting previously unresponsive patients to move, speak or dance.[77] Moreover, for older persons, the physical,

mental, and social benefits of dance can be more readily

obtained without the exertion often associated with

workouts like running or pounding the treadmill.[78]

John Zeisel, author of "I'm Still Here," and president and

co-founder of Hearthstone Alzheimer Care, believes

such alternative therapies help people with dementia

experience the essence of their lives.[79] Zeisel contends

the availability of certain basic opportunities essential

for a "life worth living while [people] are alive," such as

creativity, art, and discovery constitutes "a human

rights issue."[80] In this context, even for persons with

dementia (and especially for them), the personal agency

of participating in creative activities such as dancing,

musical performance, or art is critical to affirming the

essence of life and not losing the sense of self or

individuality.[81] As Zeisel argues, "everybody with

dementia has a lot going for them. They can experience,

they can be present, and they can develop." [82] Similarly, Donna Neuman-Bluestein, a dance therapist, maintains that even if one has dementia, Alzheimer's, or Parkinson's, they should have opportunities to move and dance because dance is a vital aspect of a life worth living.[83] According to Newman-Bluestein, the dance therapist or caregiver can be especially helpful to people with dementia who often lack the initiative to initiate movement on their own, causing them to stay frozen and sedentary.[84] As she put it, "If someone else gets them going, they can engage, and they can move a lot more... I see joy when they're moving. I see them transformed by their movement."[85] In the absence of effective pharmacological interventions, the focus should be on ensuring the optimal quality of life under the circumstances by engaging in activities that contribute to self-fulfillment, meaning, social connectedness, and even joy, despite the disease.[86]

Historically, dementia and Alzheimer's have evoked grim fear: sufferers are trapped in the shadows, their ailment often treated as a dark secret, a source of embarrassment for patients and their families. [87] In the absence of any cures, many family members and caregivers are often trapped in a vortex of frustration, bitterness, and pain as the patient's memory slips away despite best efforts. [88] As geriatrician Bill Thomas posits, the dominant narrative often seems to be that people afflicted are totally lost, stuck in "a terrible, destructive ride all the way down" till they die. [89] Thomas, who coined the phrase "tragedy narrative" to describe this perspective, is challenging people to rethink dementia and Alzheimer's care and is calling for a new and more practical approach towards the illness. [90] Likewise, Mary Fridley, the co-creator of the workshop "The Joy of Dementia, (You've Got to be Kidding)," is also urging caregivers and families to move away from "medicalizing the disease."[91] She encourages adopting a more "improvisational" flexible approach that reconceptualizes 'normal' as a coping strategy.[92] Similarly, Karen Stobbe, who spent about a third of her life as a caregiver for parents with Alzheimer's, encourages caregivers to rethink the notion of normal, to refrain from arguing or constantly saying 'no,' to abandon expectations, and to play along in the 'new normal' without judgment.[93] To be sure, such approaches may only go so far, particularly as the disease advances in severity towards the later stages. Family members dealing with the daily stress of caring for loved ones during the late stages of dementia and Alzheimer's regularly experience harrowing and unfathomable traumas with little or no support, often to the detriment of their own health, well-being, and financial security. Many caregivers describe heartbreakingly distressing episodes that push them to breaking point, including unspeakable hardships as they toil alone, sacrificing everything to care for loved ones who sometimes become very abusive, grossly indecent, and even viciously violent. [94] Quite clearly, the therapeutic dance and music interventions recommended here are likely to be more effective at ameliorating symptoms during the earlier stages. In the meantime, while we await cures for dementia and Alzheimer's, there is much that can be done to prevent, delay, or mitigate these disorders. We need to explore all viable complementary and alternative approaches to alleviate suffering, improve the quality of life, and perhaps even bring a little joyfulness for patients and their caregivers.

The push to embrace dance as complementary and alternative for neurodegenerative disorders gained momentum over the past decade as pioneering healthcare organizations and medical professionals developed innovative collaborations with dance and movement therapists, musicians, and other artists. About a decade ago, hospitals in Buenos Aires attracted global attention after they started providing therapeutic tango lessons for people suffering from neurological disorders, including Alzheimer's, Parkinson's, and depression.[95] In a landmark initiative, doctors and nurses at the Hospital de Clinicas, the country's largest psychiatric hospital, danced the tango with Parkinson's patients to help alleviate the disease's symptoms.[96] Patients who could hardly walk or stand upright took the dance floor with enthusiasm and joyfulness, dancing together, not as doctor-patient or nurse-patient, but simply as tango dancers.[97] Dr. Leticia Lopez and her colleagues observed that Parkinson's patients who regularly danced the tango experienced a slowing down symptom progression, consistent with the studies

discussed in the previous chapter.[98] Beyond managing

the disease, the dancing also provided emotional, and

other psychological benefits as patients felt supported

by medical professionals who were genuinely

committed to their well-being.[99] Lou Heber, a nursing

professor and dance therapy advocate, maintains

healing dance sessions are more effective when doctors,

nurses, or other professionals guiding the sessions also

join in.[100] As she put it, such engagement shows "you

are with the patients, not above them," building mutual

trust and making it easier for patients and caregivers to

connect.[101] Similarly, after Ukrainian doctors launched

dance classes for PD patients in 2016 collaboration

with the National Gerontology Institute and the

Ukrainian Association of Movement disorders, they

observed improvements in movement initiation,

balance, stride length, psychological well-being, and

quality of life.[102] Likewise, a small but growing number of facilities for seniors, including adult daycare and assisted living homes, have incorporated dance, movement, and music therapy as part of their dementia prevention and care programs.[103] In these interdisciplinary interventions, choreographers, dancers, and musicians collaborate with health care professionals to create little rays of light where darkness often prevails. While some programs are highly structured interventions conducted in-house, others involve partnerships with local dance instructors and studios. Moreover, these examples and anecdotes also reinforce the research findings from above: dance, movement, and music therapy can improve care and enhance the quality of life for dementia patients.

Rosener House, a unique adult daycare program in Menlo Park, California, conducted an extraordinarily engaging dance therapy program for people living with Alzheimer's, dementia, and Parkinson's to improve "cognitive function" as well as "gait and balance and spatial awareness."[104] In 2019, Rosener House administrator, Barbara Kalt, launched a therapeutic tango program dubbed "Caravan of Memory," developed by French researchers affiliated with the University of Burgundy that had previously been successfully implemented in at least eight cities around the world.[105] Troubled by the poor outcomes of current therapies and determined to transform patient care, Kalt turned to dance therapy to improve her patients' "cognition, gait and balance" or, "at the very least," make their lives "more fun and interesting." [106] Moreover, she believed that without a cure, "social interaction and physical activities are really more important" for older adults in care programs, and felt the tango therapy would reduce isolation and loneliness. [107] The dance program aligned neatly with the philosophy of her adult day care program design. Seniors who normally stayed in their homes at night could enjoy "normal social interaction" during the day, "make new friends," and enjoy a social life around eating, dining and dancing together. [108] Kalt, who believed assisted living facilities "should be the last step," felt adult daycare programs combining a healthy lifestyle and fun initiatives like tango dancing were the ideal because clients could "maintain [a] good quality of life for as long as possible."[109] Twenty-plus seniors enrolled in the program began each session with a warm-up of upper body moves, hand-clapping, and foot-stomping before beginning the tango's elegant promenade-like choreography to the sound of the bandoneon- all the while being filmed for a teachable documentary. [110] Once a week, Josh Cano, the program leader, directed participants in a simple walking dance to the music, guiding them through "steps, turns, multiple changes of partners and a water break," followed by a cool-down period with soothing piano to promote relaxation.[111] When Clarissa, the program's Argentinian instructor, asked for feedback, one man said, 'I feel that we are all just one here.' It was just so wonderful; Josh Cano, the program leader, reported beneficial "changes in people with mood, speech, and focus," and Shanah Hawk, the program coordinator, stated, "it's definitely a mood boost."[112] Kent, a participating retiree from Menlo Park, felt the program was "very subtly, but very definitely, aimed to get people active: standing up, moving, eye and hand coordination, the sense of rhythm..."[113] While conceding dancers "walk away tired and sore" and occasionally "step on a lot of feet," Kent was appreciative, stating: "There's an old saying about use it or lose it ... it's all about getting the mind working, the heart working, the enjoyment, the pleasure."[114] Even after Barbara Kalt retired, the exceptionally innovative program continued to flourish, and her "visionary" leadership continued to inspire the staff, with one current employee declaring, "Rosener House reflects her, and she is a reflection of it. Barbara just exudes this amazing light." [115] Kalt, who became a participant in the program after she retired, experienced firsthand the fruits of her handiwork. She shared the following exchange about an encounter on the dance floor: "I was dancing with a woman today, and I said, 'You have such good balance,' and she said, "Well, I learned it here."[116]

Wu Tao, which translates to "the Dancing Way," is a popular therapeutic dance intervention for people with dementia developed in 2001 by ballerina Michelle Locke.[117] Combining Chinese traditional medicine with modern techniques, Wu Tao is a tai chi style program centered on dance, music, relaxation, and meditation.[118]

Locke describes Wu Tao dance as a physical and healing workout, that is "a therapy for body and soul" comprising mostly of "gentle movement, music, and meditation" structured to harmonize the energy flow.[119] The program that uses movement to stimulate self-expression has been described as "allowing the body to be a vehicle for the soul to speak in a dance incorporating "movement and stillness, both doing and being." [120] It helps participants transcend the noise of existence and transports them to feel "the stillness of their own being," helping participants find "the ability to go with the flow of life, feeling still and ending the struggle." [121] By focusing on dance without much thought, participants are guided in a program that seeks "to restore peace, balance, and beauty to [themselves] and the world" and to "become one with the healing life force energy."[122] The Wu Tao program consists of a 25-minute choreographed dance routine consisting of five dances that balance the body by galvanizing the natural meridians or energy channels to produce a "feeling of great harmony." [123] The five dances represent the five elements that govern certain meridians or energy channels: air (lungs and large intestine), water (kidney and bladder), wood (liver and gall bladder), fire, and earth.[124] In collaboration with the Dementia Behaviour Management Advisory Service (DBMAS) and Alzheimer's Australia, researchers introduced Wu Tao dance therapy to a dementia care facility as a non-pharmacological treatment "to alleviate agitation/anxiety and promote a bond between carers and clients."[125] In a study conducted by behavior consultant Debbie Duignan, the Wu Tao psychosocial intervention reportedly helped reduce agitation and frustration in dementia patients who completed the program.[126] Participants in the dance group reported Wu Tao was a pleasurable and enjoyable therapy: 83%

agreed the dance improved their moods and made them feel happier and were agreeable to attending a session weekly in the future.[127]

At the New Courtland Life Allegheny Center in Philadelphia, dance therapist, Natasha Goldstein-Levitas, conducts a traditional hour-long dance therapy intervention for seniors with dementia and other cognitive impairments. [128] She encourages creative expression and use of movement to "unlock their potential," prompting her patients with motivational talk as needed. She also works with patients to foster their connections to society, improve quality of life, and help them to re-discover their sense of self by "stimulating reminiscence."[129] During a session, Lee Wright, a 75-year old who normally needs a cane to walk, drops it and joins 15 other residents in a circle, dancing to songs like Glenn Miller's big band classic "In

The Mood." [130] At the end of the hour, when asked how he felt, Mr. Wright proclaimed with a smile: "Some kind of wonderful." [131] Similarly, at the Arthur Murray Dance Studio in Manhattan, the instructor, Esther Frances, guides Alzheimer's patients and their caretakers to dance. [132] Eighty-year old Suzanne Paul, diagnosed with Alzheimer's, danced the Argentine tango with her seventy-seven-year-old husband, Jim Paul, both demonstrating a seriousness of purpose that impressed their instructor. [133] Like other couples in the program, Suzanne and Jim persisted through a demanding eight-week practice session that "helped improve their condition." [134] Frances also appreciates the fact that the caregivers are also catching a little break, enjoying a dance while also getting a chance to discover a glimmer of the person their patient was before being altered by the disease. [135] Meanwhile, the Alvin Ailey Dance Foundation, in partnership with the non-profit,

CaringKind, also teaches basic dance skills to help caregivers and persons with dementia "improve strength, flexibility, mobility, balance, [and] endurance. [136] The therapeutic dance program also encourages participants to explore personal stories through movement to kindle imagination and promote joy.[137] Similarly, at the Willow Towers Assisted Living Facility operated by the United Hebrew of New Rochelle, seniors, including several with dementia participate in a regular dance therapy program.[138] According to dance therapists Senta Perez-Gardner and Kelsey Gangnath, the participating seniors experience less anxiety and agitation, and dancing has improved their overall well-being and quality of life.[139]

Recall Don Henley crooning, *"Some Dance to Remember ..."* Joy Through Dance, a therapeutic dance program for residents in St. Barnabas retirement living community in the Pittsburgh area, uses music from the past to help

residents with dementia reconnect with earlier

memories of younger days, something that always gets

many to start dancing.[140] Sponsored by the St.

Barnabas Health Care System, the programmed dubbed

named "Music, Memory, and Dance," is tailored to

different levels of dementia diagnoses and provides

specially curated music playlists for each dementia

patient, based on music from their younger years. [141]

The program was inspired by Frank Glazer, senior

outreach director of the Pittsburgh Ballroom, who chose

dance and music therapy because "music is in your

head, it stays with you" forever, and listening to old

songs can literally transport a dementia patient to an

earlier, more joyful time and place. [142] The program is

supported by dancers from the Pittsburgh Ballroom and

St. Barnabas staff who work with the residents weekly

in partnership with the Alzheimer's Association -

Greater Pennsylvania Chapter. [143] The specially curated music selections motivate the residents to get up and dance with enthusiasm. One resident's spouse affirmed the program had transformed her husband, making him "more upbeat, physically and mentally."[144] Midge Hobaugh, an administrator at St. Barnabas Health System, described the program as a "perfect fit" for the facility because it brought "sheer joy" to the residents while also lessening their anxiety and increasing mobility. [145]

Dance programs that support patients with dementia are also a godsend to their caregivers. In Reno, Nevada, Donna Brown and her husband, Ron, who is living with Alzheimer's, attend Ballroom of Reno, a dementia dance therapy program run in partnership with the non-profit Dementia Friendly Washoe County.[146] After several months in the program, Ms. Brown noticed that dancing in the program produced positive behavioral changes in participants, including her husband, remarking "...everyone is happy ... [and] having a good time." [147] Her husband was quite impressed by his own transformation in the course of a few months, tooting his newfound fancy feet, stating, "For a guy that has no rhythm, turning out nice, I think."[148] Program instructor, Desiree Reid, also remarked on Ron's transformation: "His balance was getting better... And walking was getting easier. And just being jovial was easier." [149] For spouses, the program helps "bring back" partners momentarily, and enables them to build new memories going forward, despite the disease, and as a caregiving-spouse, Donna particularly appreciates the break to relax, noting "it's like you just put an hour of the disease behind." [150] Despite the burden of the disease, Ron and Donna and Ron have made dancing nearly every day a habit, with the latter observing that dancing together is "very bonding," noting that hardly a day passes without a "special touch between the two."[151]

Across the pond, Terry Hall, a 71-year old retired postal worker in Cumbria England who was diagnosed with Alzheimer's at age 67, was re-energized after "discovering the therapeutic effects of dance," while attending weekly classes as part of a dementia dance project dubbed, "Dancing Recall." [152] During dance sessions at Theatre by the Lake in Keswick, Terry enthusiastically took to the dance floor with his wife Jean, where they danced to a wide repertoire ranging from 50s pop to Pavarotti. [153] Dancing provided "a new lease of life" for Terry, affording him a fun activity he could look forward to again, especially because he no longer enjoyed his old hobbies of reading and walking after his diagnosis. [154] Besides the exercise and therapeutic benefits, Jean is grateful for the program that gives them something they can "enjoy together" as a couple, especially "the friendly, relaxed atmosphere where [they] can sing and dance together and get out of the house doing something active." [155] Daphne Cushnie, who created Dancing Recall with funding assistance from England's National Dementia Strategy, was elated by the positive outcomes. She stated, "I have always believed that dance could help people with degenerative conditions like dementia, but for many years I was a voice in the wilderness."[156] Ms. Cushnie felt that the growing support and successes of dementia dance projects like "Dancing Recall" affirmed the importance of connecting "health and social care."[157] This approach also guides the work of Dance Health Alliance, a non-profit group that supports dance interventions for patients with dementia in Queensland, Australia.[158] During a sponsored program at a nursing home for the elderly, instructor Gwen Korebrits

provided therapeutic dance lessons for residents with

dementia such as Gerda Streiner, accompanied by her

daughter Edith Streiner. [159] Ms. Streiner, who loved to

dance and was a "very good" dancer when she was

younger and married, stated she missed dancing after

her husband's death and experienced profound

loneliness.[160] Her daughter confirmed the dance

program had positively impacted her mother; she had

recovered some of her mobility and was "a lot looser in

her body motions…"[161] As the elder Ms. Streiner stated,

"I was a loner and I didn't have any movement

anymore…. [I had] nothing which I really looked

forward to, and now today, it was good."[162]

As more dance programs are being established for

dementia and Alzheimer's care, greater attention is also

being paid to the issue of inclusivity and "culturally

appropriate" interventions.[163] In light of studies suggesting that Mexican Americans may develop risk factors for Alzheimer's up to a decade earlier than others, there is a sense of great urgency.[164] To address this issue, the Latino Alzheimer's & Memory Disorders Alliance (LAMDA) launched "Bailando por la Salud" (Dancing for Health) to provide opportunities for older Latinos to enhance brain and body health.[165] The group sponsors a dance event every Saturday at Casa Maravilla, a housing development for seniors in Chicago, to encourage Latinos who are not enthused about regular exercise to get fit, as part of an effort to prevent neurodegenerative decline.[166] Whereas many of the patrons at the Casa Maravilla 'danzon' party may ordinarily find conventional exercise unappealing, they do not miss a beat as they stride to oldies but goodies, some going at it with energetic hip movements.[167] The combination of 'exercise' through dancing to familiar hits strikes the sweet spot, enabling people to get fit in a fun, comfortable, and "culturally relevant" manner while also socializing with friends and family. [168] Program instructor Juan Manuel Martínez was motivated to get involved after watching his mother suffer from Alzheimer's, stating that he was determined to do everything possible "to stay physically and mentally fit, just in case." [169] Like many caregivers of people with dementia or Alzheimer's, Veronica Cabello of Los Angeles struggled to find an affordable, high-quality adult day care facility for her 86-year old mother, Aida Arauz, that also provided "culturally appropriate" programming.[170] Eventually, Ms. Cabello found a place for her mother in UCLA's Alzheimer's and Dementia Care program that provided individually-tailored care plans, with a special focus on cultural traditions unique to each person.[171] The program also included lifestyle-enhancing benefits such as music, art, and walks in the park. From the time Ms. Arauz joined the adult daycare facility in 2012, she availed herself of the dance program, becoming "one of the favorite dancers" and inspiring other members who "feed off of her vitality." [172] As her daughter summed up the situation, "...she is the happiest now. She has a drive and thrill for life. She wants to live."[173]

*****

Accounts of patients battling Parkinson's with the help of dance and music therapists are also becoming increasingly frequent, putting a human face in front of the science but also serving as a reminder of the real pain and suffering wrought by severe neurological disorders. Viewers were amazed and overjoyed after physiotherapist Anicea Renee Gunlock of Oklahoma uploaded a video to Facebook showing Parkinson's patient, Larry Jennings, aged 73, responding to music and even dancing unassisted after a prolonged struggle with "freezing of gait."[174] After a Parkinson's patient named Alan religiously attended a weekly Dance for Parkinson's program run by the English National Ballet, there was a noticeable change in his movements. A friend observed that Alan and the others in the class could move their arms with "relative ease and control," overcoming the tremors that so often accompany the condition.[175] Meanwhile, Mary, a participant in a study about the benefits of Irish set dancing, reported dance was "definitely helping her," as evidenced in part by her increased ability to perform ordinarily routine tasks such as putting on her own shoes.[176] Similarly, after 64-year old Chicago resident Geoffrey Rodgers participated in a multi-year clinical trial involving high or moderately intense exercise for PD patients, his tremors "calmed down," with the benefits lasting for up to an hour.[177] Likewise, Eunice Benson credits the program for patients with neurodegenerative diseases at Wake Forest University for "improving her mobility and changing her life."[178] Ms. Benson, who has had Parkinson's for 15 years, stated: "I walk with a cane sometimes, but since I've been doing this [dance], I don't have to."[179] One of the researchers leading the study, Dr. Christina Hugenschmidt, shared that due to participation in the dance program, "there was increased connectivity in certain brain regions," and the outcomes "correlated with changes in balance and also decreased apathy and decreased depressive symptoms."[180] These patient stories reinforce the findings from multiple studies that demonstrate that movement and dance are indeed medicine for people with Parkinson's.

In recent years, Dance for Parkinson's has emerged as a leading force for changing how society cares for people with Parkinson's Disease. The organization was started

in 2001 by Olie Westheimer, executive director of the

Brooklyn Parkinson Group, who shared her concept of

creating a dance class for her patients with the Mark

Morris Dance Group, including co-founder David

Leventhal.[181] Westheimer wanted patients to have a

fun and positive social experience because she was

concerned that they were investing too much time

focusing on the disease and mainly looking for answers

through conventional medicine.[182] David Leventhal, one

of Westheimer's first instructors, was so inspired by the

experience that he abandoned performing to focus on

expanding the program, including through advocacy,

live-streaming classes, and developing DVDs that have

been shared with over 4,000 people worldwide.[183]

Since becoming the program director for Dance for PD,

Leventhal has provided visionary leadership for a

transformational initiative that has helped provide

relief, care, and quality of life for many patients.[184] Leventhal maintains, "Dance fits Parkinson's like a glove. Parkinson's is a multi-focal condition - it affects mood, sense of self, facial expression, mobility. Dance fits all of those…" [185] A true believer, he touts the range of mental challenges and cognitive activities entailed in dancing compared to traditional exercises such as bike riding or weightlifting.[186] For example, when dancing, he observed, "You are constantly thinking about patterns, and it involves memory and problem-solving," as well as "weight shifting and balance transferring," benefits that make it a "very sophisticated movement." [187] David Leventhal would also like to see patients move beyond looking at dance therapy as merely exercising; he seeks to help patients rebuild the bridge between body and brain by incorporating an "artistic element," including stimulating music.[188] Dance for PD works with professional dance instructors like Kate

Mitchell, who leverage their expertise to engage patients through dance, while also enhancing their mobility, independence, and quality of life.[189] Mitchell, who prepared for her role by educating herself about the nature, causes, and progression of the disease, stated: "Dance for PD is not about precision or correctness [as in conventional dance programs], it's about finding joy" through movement. [190] Thus, Stanford University's Dance for PD program considers its class "a group artistic experience" that combines social and classic dance elements with live music, poetry, and imagery to motivate participants to engage in creative movements.[191] Program instructor, Damara Ganley, trains patients "to be in their bodies in a conscious way," employing a range of interactive approaches that inspire patients to engage their bodies in creative ways, including stretching, "extension and flexibility and moving with intention."[192] In one class, she ignites a kinetic conversation, encouraging participants to each "say something with the body" to another in a circle 'dance,' a process repeated with different partners, stimulating an interactive improvisational iteration that fosters creativity. [193] She mixes things up, combining simple gestures that express specific sentiments such as gratitude before transitioning to a delightful and inspirational traditional Israeli circle dance with a series of steps that require focused concentration. [194] Similarly, working with the co-founders of the Parkinson's Dance Project (Joanabbey Sack and Sarah Humphrey), choreographer Sylvain Emard teaches dance physiotherapy for Parkinson's using elaborate expansive movements in an approach called "BIG." [195] Patients were encouraged to point in the air with their arms with a "big gesture" that "builds on the aptitude" of the patient's movement, "opening your arms really wide, taking large steps, standing up straight" – an approach "focusing on increasing amplitude, on repetition, and on brain plasticity."[196] Neurologist Dr. Neil Mahant, of Sydney's Westmead Hospital, stated that such "exaggerated [dance] movements" can help Parkinson's patients overcome issues related to scale of movement. [197] In effect, practicing "larger movements in class can carry through into daily life" and "high intensity and exaggerated activities could improve symptoms" by helping patients whose movements are severely constricted to expand their range.[198] While the tango appears to be a popular choice in many Parkinson's dance programs, some experts are concerned that the tango's complex and highly structured movements may be too much for some patients.[199] In an endeavor that could address this challenge, David Leventhal has partnered with Dr. Pietro Mazzoni, associate professor of neurology at Washington University in St. Louis, to develop a basic "walking dance," consisting of a brief warm-up followed by a structured and expressive walk.[200] Mazzoni, who plans to study the effects of dancing on Parkinson's patients, believes the simple choreography helps isolate moves that are most beneficial for Parkinson's patients. He suggests the program can help free patients constricted patterns by opening up a "broader range of movement possibilities, teaching their brains to respond in new ways, forming new neural pathways."[201]

In account shared by Gail Kent in the Virginian-Pilot, dancing has made a big difference in the life of her husband Bob Kent, and several others who suffer from Parkinson's Disease.[202] Bob, aged 76, and Gail enjoy dancing the rhumba and other genres at Two Left Feet Dance Studio for Alzheimer's and Parkinson's patients in Hampton Roads, Virginia, under the guidance of instructors Rick Tvelia and Lin Hines.[203] The couple, who met four decades earlier while disco dancing at a Parks and Recreation class in Newport News, frequently enjoyed dancing together when they were younger, but "after marriage and children, … dancing was relegated to the occasional wedding or corporate event." [204] Following Bob's diagnosis over a decade ago, medications gave him some respite from his symptoms for a while; however, the disease progressively "hampered his movement, distorted his gait, sapped his energy and wounded his confidence." [205] After agreeing to try the dancing class, Bob was quickly transformed into an aficionado. He stuck with the program, "even on 'bad' days," and attested to its benefits, stating: "The class makes me get out of the house and forces me to move even when I don't feel like it, which is most of the time, … I would be self-conscious in a regular class where I would stand out as someone with limited movement, but since everyone has Parkinson's, I don't worry about the way I look and move."[206]   Gail wrote

she did not need a study to validate the program's

impact. She declared the program was "medicine for

both of us, giving us something to focus on besides the

disease progression," replacing "some of the quality of

life we lost," including the joy of "reconnecting" as a

couple affectionately.[207] Gail added that the dance

program positively impacted their friends, Kathi Griffin,

a retired minister, and her husband LeRoy Griffin, also a

retired minister and accountant, who was diagnosed

with Parkinson's about five years earlier.[208] Following

his doctor's recommendation, the seventy-four-year-old

Mr. Griffin ramped up exercise, including dance,

resulting in positive self-assessments about his balance

and coordination. [209] Reflecting on his progress, Mr.

Griffin stated, "I do think I feel a little smoother in some

of my movements... And my serve toss while playing

tennis seems to be a little better than I remember it

being last fall."[210] Mr. Griffin has also improved in coordinating and executing his dance moves when he spins his wife on the dance floor, noting, "My left arm is no longer — as (my wife) Kathi says — taking her head off when we do turns."[211] Kathi, who had primarily viewed PD "as such a debilitating thing," could now "reframe," stating, "...that's why the dancing is so much fun... It's one of the few things we do that's just our time... to be able to dance and have fun puts the disease in a whole different category."[212]

In an article in Stanford Medicine in Winter 2017, Ruth Ann Richter wrote about the transformations experienced by several Parkinson's patients in the university's dance program, the brainchild of neuroscientist Helena Bronte-Stewart and her colleagues.[213] Sherry Brown, 74, diagnosed with PD in 2008, was one of 20 patients who joined the dance classes every Monday and Friday at the Stanford Neuroscience Center, fulfilling the founders' vision of a program that had community engagement as a key focus. [214] When first diagnosed, she despaired her "life was over;" as the disease symptoms progressed, her balance worsened, leading to injurious falls. She has experienced some physical improvement following a treatment regimen that is complemented by lifestyle interventions, including fitness training, daily walks, and participating in Stanford's Dance for PD. [215] Dancing to music, like a key, helps unlock some of the stiffness created by PD, enabling her to open her arms "in a wide, upward arc," to push her "body to do things" she did not think were achievable.[216] The combination of dancing and music produces "subtle" but impactful changes: the rhythm "helps keep things" like gait "more even," and her "body feels more in tune – more rhythmic," and she leaves the sessions "feeling energized and relaxed...and ready to move."[217] Moreover, dancing provides a psychological boost and lessens her fear of "the unknown;" it increases her sense of agency in both "big and little things" - enabling her to "adjust to the future," while keeping focus "on the here and now." [218] She feels that by combining her medications with exercise and dance, she is "definitely delaying the severe symptoms of the disease," and she is "determined to do what she can to forestall any further physical decline" and "to stay in the present" as much as possible. [219]

It should be clear by now that you do not need fancy feet to avail yourself of the dance cure. Cori Coble, who held a free dance therapy class at Jacksonville University for people with PD, invited everyone to participate, stating, "Everybody has the right to dance, everybody should be able to dance...You don't have to be good at it. You just have to enjoy it."[220]   While certain

dance steps can be challenging for some patients, dance

therapist/tango teacher Charlotte Millour maintained

that there are added therapeutic benefits when people

take the initiative to get up and dance in social settings.

[221] For example, tango dance therapy facilitates the

"encounter and exchange" between two persons; as

they move towards each other in unison with focused

eye contact, patients experience an increased sense of

connectedness and vitality.[222] Suppose tango dancing or

swing does not work for you, not to worry. Pick your

poison or potion from a broad palate: you can try

square dancing, hip-hop dancing, or even Zumba, the

popular craze that has also been shown to alleviate the

symptoms of neurodegenerative decline.[223] Regardless

of the genre, the key is to get up and get moving and to

work with your physician and dance therapist to

develop an individually-tailored regimen appropriate

for your condition. As Dr. Mary Tinetti, chief of geriatrics at the Yale University School of Medicine, observed, many dances appear to help address motor coordination and balance challenges for dementia and Parkinson's patients, including "culturally specific" genres, such as African dancing or folk dancing.[224]

*****

In the absence of cures, music therapy is also emerging as an effective alternative and or complementary treatment to lessen the suffering and trauma associated with neurodegenerative diseases like dementia, Alzheimer's, and Parkinson's.[225] Writing in the Boston Globe, Karen Weintraub declared music therapy "today's cutting-edge Alzheimer's treatment" because it provides some relief to patients, helping them express themselves creatively, and develop stronger connections with others.[226] Thus, during music therapy class at Hebrew Senior Life's NewBridge on the Charles campus, three women bonded by performing together, transcending the isolation that often attends dementia: Carla and Dorothy played the tambourine and xylophone respectively, while Leni tapped on an African drum. [227]   Others joined in by singing and dancing to an old Doris Day hit without any prompting - the music serving as a catalyst to unlock the creative spirit inside as they all performed together – a consequential development because many dementia and Alzheimer's patients have difficulty expressing themselves and making connections with other people. [228] These programs can also help reduce some of the behavioral challenges, such as agitation and anxiety, associated with dementia. For example, David Kaplan of Waltham, Massachusetts, shared that art classes in the NewBridge memory care unit were a "calming influence" for his wife, Nancy, a resident.[229] At a

Marlborough, Massachusetts, home for 45 people with

dementia, music therapist Joshua Freitas'

performances were a soothing influence, dramatically

reducing the agitation that was otherwise typical among

most residents in the evenings and possibly obviating

the need for tranquilizers.[230] Diana K. Miller, program

manager for a residential facility housing dementia

patients, observed that relying on "music and art, and

movements," and not just on verbal skills, helps

dementia patients thrive because the "primary language

is emotion." [231] These and previous examples show once

again that residents with dementia or Alzheimer's

benefit greatly when program administrators like those

at Hearthstone facilities in Massachusetts implement

creative alternative therapies involving art, music and

dance. For example, one resident's daughter in

Englewood, NJ wrote, "My mother was given the

priceless gift of reconnecting with the part of her that is

and always will be a musician. Seeing my mother's true spirit come back to life, and shine through her eyes that day she began to play music again was an experience I will never forget."[232] Another person in Maryland shared that when her relative arrived at the Hearthstone residence "in a wheelchair, she was unable to walk or feed herself," but, a few weeks later, "On our visits, she ... sang and danced freely," was able to walk independently with little or no assistance..."[233] In a comment to the Boston Globe, Jen Hayward wrote, "Music and art are wonderful for those with Alzheimer's ... I have seen the benefits for a relative in our family. It is a transformation to joy that we never expected but for which are eternally grateful!"[234]

We all know listening to just the right piece of music can be a very uplifting experience, as music can help revive happy memories and spur a cathartic journey down memory lane, something we all need from time to time. For people with dementia, music can have a potent therapeutic effect. Enjoying a favorite piece of music has been shown to trigger short and long term memory in patients at the early stages of dementia, helping some recall and relive forgotten experiences.[235] Marian Brown, associate director of Artz: Artists for Alzheimer's, told a story about a dementia patient who was transported to the happy summers of her teen years when she listened to music by Frank Sinatra.[236] In that case, the music was "very clearly something that triggered a deep-rooted memory," revealing long-term memories and emotions are quite present and alive, despite the cognitive decline that comes with Alzheimer's.[237] Studies also show that dementia patients treated with music therapy needed less antidepressant and antipsychotic drugs, which some experts contend are too liberally prescribed.[238] Playlist for Life, an English charity that curates personal playlists for people with dementia, achieved a 60 percent reduction in the use of psychotropic medication at a nursing home for participating patients, and the patients also exhibited less agitation.[239] Policymakers are taking note. Troubled by the "over-medicalisation and dishing out pills when it's not in the best interests of the [dementia] patient..." Matt Hancock, the U.K.'s Minister of Health, announced the government's commitment to "personalized care" alternatives that use music to help reduce agitation and bring calm to people with dementia.[240] To support caregivers working with music therapy, the Mayo Clinic provides the following guidelines to help those using to help a loved one with Alzheimer's disease.[241] Caregivers and therapists should select music consistent with the person's preferences, especially music that can spark memories of happy times, and not hesitate to replay favorites. In that regard, it is advisable to use appropriate music to "set the mood," play a soothing melody to promote calm or something upbeat, and faster-paced to help elevate mood. [242] For example, it is recommended that caregivers avoid music that leads to adverse reactions and any competing sounds such as television that could overstimulate and trigger confusion. [243] Caregivers or therapists should encourage singing along, tapping to the beat, or even dancing together where appropriate or possible.[244] Some therapists have also suggested a form of silent dance as an appropriate form of musical therapy for dementia and Alzheimer's. [245] Silent dances or silent discos were first popularized by young people at music festivals who donned wireless headphones that piped music directly to their ears, rather than a loudspeaker. [246] Some caregivers have found that certain shy seniors respond more favorably to silent dance therapy, enabling them to sing and dance on their own in greater comfort.[247] Australia's Move & Groove, founded by Alison Harrington, with funding support from the NSW government, also uses senior silent disco dance to help seniors with dementia; the group has partnered with dance therapists and operates in Sydney, Melbourne, and the UK.[248]

*****

Over the years, as evidence of its efficacy mounted, dance therapy in the United States overcame many barriers and gained greater acceptance. Health organizations are increasingly moving past the history of skepticism and suspicion and developing partnerships between physicians and dance therapists, and other artists. For example, some doctors who have collaborated with therapists to care for Parkinson's patients have found an eye-opening experience; many concede they have gained fresh and valuable insights.[249]

After working with Sarah Robichaud, a former dancer

who runs a free dance for Parkinson's program in

Toronto, Dr. Metlof became more convinced of the

therapeutic benefits of dance.[250] Likening his patients'

transformation to a transcendence, he observed that not

every solution to the disease is found in a bottle of

pills.[251] Neurologist Dr. Nabila Dahodwala of

Pennsylvania Hospital, who has also worked with dance

therapists, has been similarly pleased with patient

feedback from dance interventions.[252] She shared that

after participating in the program, patients state "they

feel empowered" and are "so grateful" to regain control

over their bodies and to move to music again, skills they

believed they had lost completely.[253] Such successes led

Dr. Jay van Gerpen, a neurologist at Mayo Clinic's

campus in Jacksonville, to remark that he is "very

enamored" with dance as a therapeutic intervention for

managing PD because the patients have better functional outcomes with dancing that helps improve their balance - with the added bonus of being a fun and sociable activity. [254] The possibility of integrating dance therapists into improved patient care for dementia and Parkinson's is opening up new opportunities to combine the best of modern medicine with the arts, specifically music and dance. As these examples illustrate, therapeutic dance is gradually emerging as a viable, alternative, and a complementary option for patients afflicted by neurological disorders. Since we have not yet found cures for diseases such as Alzheimer's, Parkinson's, and dementia, these non-pharmacological options should be prioritized and leveraged to improve patient care. Quite clearly, guided therapeutic interventions, movement, exercise, dance, and music therapy can contribute to positive health outcomes and, at a minimum, enhance the quality of life.

The Ancient and Modern Healing Art of Dance

In many respects, contemporary DMT connects the best of all worlds, combining ancient practices such as tai chi with modern scientific approaches, blending the healing arts with the new science and technology of medicine. [255] As dance therapy has gained respectability worldwide, the number of such innovations is growing, including innovative variations that borrow from various global tributaries, as illustrated below. As discussed above, music, dance, and singing were central components of the ancient world's healing ceremonies and rituals. However, advances in contemporary science and technology relegated the healing arts to the background, solidifying the triumphant surge of medical science.[256] Moreover, jealously guarding their ascendant status, western medical professionals were initially very skeptical, perhaps even territorial, as they walled off the new science of medicine from the healing arts.[257] As the 'cold war' thaws, dance therapists are increasingly collaborating with practitioners of the science of medicine, closing the gap and mending the rift between the healing arts and modern medicine. [258] In a creative convergence of diverse streams, tai chi, yoga dance, qi gong, mindful movement, and other ancient practices are increasingly interwoven with contemporary wellness programs to improve physical and mental health.[259] Queensland dance therapist, Yumi Schaefer, thinks this meeting of worlds is an "inspirational movement" because it brings together diverse approaches from global dance cultures and creates alternative pathways to health and happiness. [260] As dance therapy enters the mainstream, these diverse intercultural dance experiences could be leveraged to offer relief to patients with neurodegenerative disorders. Moreover, as stated earlier, novelty (as in new and different dances) is particularly beneficial for sustaining brain health.

In an exciting confluence of cultural streams, new hybrid forms of therapeutic dance are increasingly common in wellness regimens. Thus, Harris Eyre and his colleagues noted the growing popularity in the West of yoga and other ancient Eastern mind-body interventions such as tai chi, mindfulness meditation, and qi gong.[261] This trend is benefitting from studies showing that combining movement or dance with the meditation and mindfulness practices associated with yoga creates more beneficial health impacts.[262] Meanwhile, Neuromuscular Integrative Action (NIA), a yoga-dance routine dubbed "the dance of joy" by Yoga Journal, is an exciting hybrid approach that combines an organized yoga workout, dance, and elements of martial arts.[263] In Nepal, dance therapist Kamala Neupane established the first of its kind School of Dance Therapy, combining traditional yoga-style breathing and stretching techniques with dance movements to address ailments such as neurological disorders, diabetes, and hypertension.[264] Meanwhile, tantrum yoga was introduced in Los Angeles-based yoga teacher Hemalayaa. [265] Practitioners vent frustrations and anxieties and exorcise demons by screaming, shaking, dancing, and engaging in traditional yoga asanas with breathing and meditation exercises.[266] Elsewhere, some have found solace in popular yoga raves that originated in Argentina before spreading to several countries. [267] Practitioners typically start with conventional stretches, breathing, meditation, and transcendence before culminating in high-energy dance parties. [268] Those seeking something very different have turned to twerking yoga; developed by New York-based yoga instructor Barbara Purcell, the regimen involves activating the lower chakra with a slight, sexually charged twerk.[269]

Pioneering dance therapists in India also blend old and new as they leverage the country's rich heritage, developing programs that use great classical dances, including the Bharatanatyam, Kathak, Manipuri, Kuchipudi, as well as martial dances like Chau and Paika.[270] The Bharatanatyam, especially, is a popular choice for contemporary Indian practitioners because of certain elements, including its "yogic postures" that make it uniquely suited for therapeutic dance interventions.[271] For example, during the Bharatanatyam's basic stance of araimandi (a squat in which knees are turned sideways), performers are expected to keep the torso steady while the hands and lower limbs move. [272] This intricate maneuver helps with balance, imagination, and memory, requiring performers to remember very long sequences and seamlessly improvise when memory fails. [273] Moreover, the elegant Bharatanatyam also requires high levels of coordination with highly complex yogic poses and elaborate hand and finger movements (mudras) such as the chinhamudra and Hamsasyam. [274] As noted earlier, such mentally testing dances can help enhance the brain's neuroplasticity and stave off neurodegenerative decline. Thus, Geeta Chandra, a teacher and dance therapist, observed that the Bharatanatyam is particularly appropriate for helping patients achieve cathartic release and de-stress because it demands such a high level of focus.[275] At India's Srishti Institute of Dance Therapy, instructors integrate the Bharatanatyam into a holistic healing program for patients with mental and physical ailments.[276] The

Institute combines contemporary techniques with the Bharatanatyam's elegance and vitality to provide a unique psycho-therapeutic process based on connecting mind, body, and spirit as part of the healing process.[277] Similarly, in Bangalore, Odissi teacher, Jigisha Roy Majumda, runs a dance program for women middle-aged women with neurological disorders that reportedly achieved positive results, including several participating patients who made remarkable recoveries.[278] Despite its reported effectiveness, the Bharatanatyam is an unusually challenging dance for novices, prompting some dance therapists to modify it for the students. For example, Chennai based Mala Bharath, founded the Athma Laya or 'inner harmony' dance therapy program for women, based on a less strict version of the Bharatanatyam.[279] The program provides an opportunity for women who are experiencing stress to revitalize themselves while listening to great Sanskrit works like Soundarya Lahari and Indian poets such as Mahakavi Bharathiyar and Arunachala Kavirayar.[280] Similarly, Tripura Kashyap developed a less rigid and contemporary approach to the intricate and demanding mudras of Bharatanatyam and Chau for her students. [281] In a hybrid program that primarily uses soothing instrumental music from Africa and Asia, Kashyap has built a unique practice for corporate clientele who have reported they developed greater confidence and other useful business skills.[282] It is also thought that the Bharatanatyam improves blood circulation, particularly from the fingers to the rest of the body, helping to soothe the mind, aid rehabilitation, strength conditioning, and overall mental health.[283] Meanwhile, Amar Agarwal, an Indian ophthalmologist, also suggests that the Bharatanatyam improves vision because it provides eye muscles a substantial workout as dancers adroitly roll their eyes from side to side, communicating various messages. [284] Furthermore,

many Indian dance therapy practitioners combine

movement with mindfulness and meditation,

incorporating yoga moves associated with the Bhagavad

Gita's three pathways to self-realization (Bhakti, Jnana,

or Karma) into their choreographies.[285]

Less structured but equally therapeutic, ecstatic healing

dance circles are thriving around the U.S. with

structured as well as informal programs. Participants

who are sometimes referred to as trance,

improvisational or spontaneous dancers typically chant,

drum, sing, and dance in 'tribes' where they find

solidarity, social connectedness as well as physical,

emotional, and spiritual benefits. [286] In the 5Rhythms

movement, a more structured program, there is an

elaborate meditation framework where participants

move through each phase with a different intention,

gaining awareness of how energy courses through their bodies. [287] Sonya Pritzker, a Chinese medicine practitioner and assistant professor of anthropology at the University of Alabama who runs a monthly dance "tribe" in Tuscaloosa, found ecstatic dances produce emotional and spiritual benefits. [288] Her students reported that trance dancers experienced freedom from anxiety, negative thoughts, and stress while also enjoying the freedom to "move without constraints, be present, connect with others or experience joy – and pain" together as a tribe.[289] Commenting her lived experience in the Times, Tam Hunt called "ecstatic dance [her] religion ... [and] Hippy church" and described the worldwide "ecstatic dance movement" as a "really beneficial new phenomenon for health and longevity." [290] Meanwhile, Synergy Dance developed an approach, based on polarity therapy principles and the five elements (earth, water, fire, air, and ether), to use healing energy to free the spirit through self-expressive movement.[291] Participants seek to achieve holistic body and spirit fitness by combining physical, mental, and spiritual approaches sourced from diverse cultures and traditions, including sacred circle dancing, African dance, Indian dance, Turkish belly dancing, and yoga. [292] In the same intercultural vein, Marsha Scarbrough, author of *Medicine Dance*, built a unique healing arts practice that combines her experiences with Native American, African and Asian traditions. [293] Leveraging her experiential training in dance therapy, Buddhist meditation, martial arts as well as Native American and West African spirituality, she helps clients find healing and peace through workshops such as Shaman's Barefoot Disco and participation in sweat lodges, African drumming, meditations, and dance fasts. [294] Similarly, Eileen Fairbane borrowed from diverse intercultural streams to create the Fairbane Method, an alternative dance intervention to ward off illness by treating the whole person. [295] The approach combines Native American, Asian, and Chakra dancing with hands-on bodywork (aromatherapy, massage oils) and a psychological workout focusing on the chakras, counseling, breathing, visualization, meditation, nutrition, and herbal supplements.[296]

In a New Agey approach to therapeutic dance, Rolando Toro Araneda, a Chilean psychologist and medical anthropologist, developed an interdisciplinary program called Biodanza or *Life Dance.*[297] The program encourages reflection, movement, and lots of dancing and hugging to increase self-knowledge in five areas of human potential or "Vivencias" - vitality, sexuality, creativity, affectivity, and transcendence.[298] The multidisciplinary program that unites "art, science, and love" draws from physiology, psychology, and biology, emphasizing how one's personal ecology or environment, and the quality of interactions or relations therein, determines one's potential. [299] In programs such as "dancing the archetypes of joy, sensuality, and wellbeing," participants experienced the benefits of dancing in an environment filled with like-minded positive people to enhance feelings of well-being, connectedness, and happiness.[300] An assessment by Marcus Stueck at the University of Leipzig in Germany showed Biodanza sessions had demonstrably a positive mental health impact on participants. [301] Stueck found that after ten weekly Biodanza sessions, participants were more relaxed and hopeful, demonstrated better anger management skills, displayed improved interpersonal and problem-solving skills, and had more robust immune systems.[302]

Other pioneers are experimenting with new hybrid approaches that combine modern dance clubs or gyms with elements of therapeutic dance including, wellness programs, trained instructors, dance therapists, and professional dancers. For example, neuroscientist and researcher Dr. Rehfeld seeks to leverage her research findings in a commercialized dance and mental fitness and wellness program called 'Jymmin,' (jamming and gymnastic).[303] Emphasizing fitness programs that can maximize anti-aging effects on the brain, the 'Jymmin' approach is a sensor-based system that generates rhythms and melodies in response to physical activity.[304] Meanwhile, dance entrepreneur Sadie Kurzban launched 305 Fitness, a popular Miami nightclub-style dancercise dance party that she claims combines the fun of dance with a workout.[305] Similarly, Daybreaker holds early morning dancercise workouts based on community values and experiences such as wellness, self-expression, and mindfulness.[306]

Combining working out with wellness, mindfulness, and yoga with the help of professional instructors and dance therapists in a typical night club (without alcohol) could be an appealing way to introduce a new generation to the social, mental, and physical benefits of ancient healing dances.[307] As a sign of how far things have come, dance therapy made its cyberspace debut after a pioneering app was created by UC Irvine graduate student Kate Ringland, and her team, for Kinect.[308] The dance therapy app challenged students to mimic dance moves next to cartoon-like characters on the console, helping players gain greater awareness of their bodies.[309]

VI. One More Thing: An Ounce of Preventive Lifestyle Medicine

Without question, movement, exercise, and dance have significant therapeutic effects, including positive neurological, physiological, and psychological impacts. As demonstrated above, movement, exercise, and dance could help prevent or delay the onset of neurological disorders and serve as complementary therapies for those receiving treatment for these disorders. To be sure, for those suffering from neurological disorders, dance and movement therapy would not solve the underlying disease. It is a tragedy that we have not yet found a way to cure dementia, Alzheimer's, and Parkinson's. Going forward, significant changes in public policy, including massive hikes in research funding and entrepreneurial 'moonshot' initiatives, are in order. Given the projected increases in these disorders in the years ahead, there is grave urgency. We all know someone who has dementia, Alzheimer's, Parkinson's, depression, and other mood disorders. Each one of us could be the next victim of these punishing diseases. In the absence of cures, prevention is paramount. While movement-exercise and dance are by no means cures for these cruel diseases, they provide needed relief for many patients. It is recommended that people who are already struggling with dementia, Alzheimer's, or dementia work with a dance therapist or other health professional to implement appropriate regimens. As noted earlier, even where appropriate, these alternative or complementary therapies may be most effective at the earlier stages of neurodegenerative disorders.

While lifestyle prescriptions about physical activity, sleep, or nutrition may be of little or no value at advanced stages of disease, they are a major difference-maker when implemented early on. Therefore, make physical activity part of your daily life by combining conventional exercise with rhythmic movement, music, and dance. In particular, to forestall neurodegenerative decline that results in dementia, Alzheimer's, and Parkinson's, the prescription here (as in my other books on preventive health) urges all exercisers to make dancing a component of their regimen.[1] As discussed earlier, dancing to music more so than other physical activities is an unusually "potent cocktail" with wide-ranging physiological, psychological, emotional, and neurological impacts.[2] Your uniquely tailored combination of movement, exercise, and dance can be designed around one of five dosage levels described below, consistent with your needs, capabilities, and health goals.

(1) The highest dose is 420 minutes weekly of moderately intense movement, exercise, and dance, or 210 minutes of vigorous intensity to maximize preventive health and longevity benefits. At this level of commitment, you are investing about 30 to 60 minutes every day of the week to achieve very substantial and wide-ranging preventive health goals and increasing your likelihood of healthy longevity.

(2) The second option consists of 360 minutes weekly of moderately intense movement, exercise, and dance. Alternatively, you can choose 180 minutes of vigorous intensity. This dosage requires you to dedicate about 30 to 60 minutes, six days a week to achieve your preventive health goals and increase your chances of healthy aging.

(3) The third option is 300 minutes weekly of moderately intense movement, exercise, and dance; or, you may opt for 150 minutes of vigorous intensity. This dosage calls for a commitment of 30 to 60 minutes, five days a week, to achieve your preventive health goals and increase your likelihood of healthy longevity.

(4) This mid-range dosage comprises 240 minutes weekly of moderately-intense movement, exercise, and dance; or, you may opt for 120 minutes of vigorous-intensity. This dosage requires a commitment of about 30 to 60 minutes, four days a week, to achieve your preventive health goals, preventive health goals, and increase your likelihood of healthy longevity.

(5) This minimum recommended dose consists of 180 minutes weekly of moderately- intense movement, exercise, and dance; or, you may choose 90 minutes of

vigorously-intensity. This dosage requires a commitment of about 30 to 60 minutes three days a week to achieve your preventive health goals, including reducing the likelihood of chronic illness and extending your life.

In choosing the dosage that is right for you should review your specific life situation and health goals, taking into account the risks of insufficient inactivity and relevant health risks as assessed by your health care professional. Moderately intense physical activity is envisioned as moving rapidly enough to burn 3-6 times more energy compared to when sedentary. This may include such activities as brisk walking, gardening, and dancing, as you work up a little sweat, pump up your heart rate and feel a little out of breath. Vigorous physical activity entails a higher degree of strenuous intensity as typical in activities such as running, swimming laps, bicycling at least ten mph, and aerobic dancing. To maximize the benefits, dance or rhythmic movement should equate to at least a third of your weekly physical activity. Furthermore, it is recommended that you allocate some time daily for mindfulness meditation, reflection, and rest. Regardless of the option selected, you should turbo-charge the benefits making other lifestyle modifications as needed, including key areas such as appropriate nutrition, tobacco avoidance, moderation in alcohol, good sleep habits, social connectedness, and environmental compatibility. Of course, you can adjust your dosage and incorporate other lifestyle modifications as your needs and circumstances change.

Although the recommended dosages exceed the standard federal exercise guidelines, they are consistent with research findings that suggest we need much more exercise than recommended in the current guidelines. [3] For example, in two articles published on the issue of 'how much exercise,' I-Min Lee and her colleagues have shown that at about an hour daily is just about right to reduce all-cause mortality.[4] Nonetheless, even if you cannot achieve the higher recommended dosages, you should strive to incorporate as much movement into your daily activities because research shows as little as 7-10 daily could be a difference-maker.[5]

Fun is a crucial element of this prescription for movement, exercise, and dance. Transform your regimen into an opportunity for social engagement with family and friends. If you walk, find suitable nature trails or scenic walkways. Infuse music and dance into as many daily activities as possible. With joyful music and dancing at least a third of your regimen, make your 'workout' a time for gain without pain. Be sure to refresh constantly, with new music and new dances, perhaps even in new locales. Infuse uplifting songs, music, and dance into your daily routines. As centenarian Clare Willis, who danced continuously for decades, put it, "You can dance every motion in your life... Every motion you do, you can turn into a dance..."[6] One more thing, to quote the memorable Steve Jobs. I hope you dance ... I hope you remember that you, yes, you too, you are an "athlete of God." I hope you feel the ethereal union of mind-body-spirit as you experience the "mysterious" music and dance of the universe and its killer riffs courtesy of the "Invisible Piper."[7]

*****

ENDNOTES

Chapter I

[1] Kaleah McIlwain, *Dance for Health*, Penn Memory Center, https://pennmemorycenter.org/programs-services/dance-for-health/.

[2] *Id.*

[3] *Id.*

[4] *Id.*

[5] *Id.*

[6] *Id.*

[7] *Id.*

[8] *Id.*

[9] *Id.*

[10] *Id.*

[11] *Id.*

[12] *Id.*

[13] Danielle Kennedy, *Reflection: West Philadelphia Seniors Bond in PMC Dance for Health program*, Sept. 18, 2018, https://pennmemorycenter.org/reflection-west-philadelphia-seniors-bond-in-pmc-dance-for-health-program/.

[14] *Id.*

[15] *Id.*

[16] *Id.*

[17] *Id.*

[18] Kaleah McIlwain, *supra* note 1. Danielle Kennedy, *supra* note 13.

[19] Ruth A. Richter, A New Rhythm, Dance Benefits Parkinson's Patients, Stanford Medicine, Winter 2017, http://stanmed.stanford.edu/2017winter/dance-for-parkinsons-disease-at-the-stanford-neuroscience-health-center.html

[20] World Health Organization, *Neurological Disorders, Public Health Challenges*, 2006. https://www.who.int/mental_health/neurology/neurodiso/en/.

[21] *Id.*

[22] Mayo Clinic, Dementia, Overview, https://www.mayoclinic.org/diseases-conditions/dementia/symptoms-causes/syc-20352013. World Health Organization *supra* 20. *See generally*, National Institute on Aging, NIH, *What Causes Alzheimer's Disease?* https://www.nia.nih.gov/health/what-causes-alzheimers-

disease. NIH, *Alzheimer's Disease, Genetics Fact Sheet*, https://www.nia.nih.gov/health/alzheimers-disease-genetics-fact-sheet; WebMD, *Causes of Alzheimer's Disease*, https://www.webmd.com/alzheimers/guide/alzheimers-causes-risk-factors; CDC, *Alzheimer's and Related Dementias*, https://www.cdc.gov/features/alzheimers-disease-dementia/index.html. *Quick Facts,* Alzheimer's Association, https://www.alz.org/alzheimers-dementia/facts-figures. Kathleen Fifield, *AARP, Dementia vs. Alzheimer's: Which Is It?* June 25, 2018. Alzheimer's Association, *Treatments for Behavior*, https://alz.org/alzheimers-dementia/treatments/treatments-for-behavior. *See also, Blood Flow to Brain Linked to Dementia*, https://www.webmd.com/heart-disease/news/20050830/blood-flow-to-brain-linked-to-dementia; Society of Nuclear Medicine, *Brain Blood Flow Gives Clues to Treating Depression*, Science Daily, Aug. 14, 2007, https://www.sciencedaily.com/releases/2007/08/070808132027.htm. Newsmax Health, *Study: Brain Blood Flow Affects Parkinson's Risk*, Newsmax, 31 Aug. 2019, https://www.newsmax.com/health/health-news/brain-blood-stroke-parkinsons/2019/08/31/id/930717/.

[23] *Id.*

[24] *Id.* See also, Margaret Gatz el al, *"Education and the Risk of Alzheimer's Disease: Findings from the Study of Dementia in Swedish Twins,"* The Journal of Gerontology: Series B, Vol. 56:5, Sept. 1, 2001, pp. 292–300. WHO *supra* note 20. *See generally,* supra note 22.

[25] See generally, *supra* note 22. WHO *supra* note 20.

[26] *Id.*

[27] *Id.*

[28] *Id.*

[29] *Id.*

[30] Cyrus R.A et al. *"Longitudinal Relationships between Caloric Expenditure and Gray Matter in the Cardiovascular Health Study." Journal of Alzheimer's disease* vol. 52,2 (2016).

[31] *Id.*

[32] Johns Hopkins, Health, *Blood Pressure and Alzheimer's Risk: What's the Connection?* https://www.hopkinsmedicine.org/health/conditions-and-diseases/alzheimers-disease/blood-pressure-and-alzheimers-risk-whats-the-connection. *Blood Flow to Brain Linked to Dementia, supra* note 22. Society of Nuclear Medicine, *supra* note 22. Newsmax Health, *supra* note 22.

[33] Zheng, F. et al, *HbA1c, Diabetes and Cognitive Decline: The English Longitudinal Study of Ageing*, Diabetologia, (2018) 61. Nicholas

Bakalar, *High Blood Sugar Levels Tied to Memory Decline*, N.Y Times, Feb. 12, 2018.

[34] *Id.*

[35] *Id.* Olga Khazan, *The Startling Link Between Sugar and Alzheimer's*, The Atlantic, Jan. 26, 2018. Harvard Mahoney Neuroscience Institute, *Sugar and the Brain*, https://neuro.hms.harvard.edu/harvard-mahoney-neuroscience-institute/brain-newsletter/and-brain/sugar-and-brain

[36] *Id.*

[37] *Id.*

[38] *Id.*

[39] Judith Graham, *Does Depression Contribute to Dementia?* N.Y. Times, May 1, 2013. Andrea Petersen, *New Therapies Help Patients with Dementia Cope with Depression*, N.Y. Times, Dec. 8, 2019.

[40] Diniz, B.S, et al, *Late-life Depression and Risk of Vascular Dementia and Alzheimer's disease: Systematic review and Meta-analysis of Community-based Cohort Studies*, British J. of Psychiatry, vol. 202, no. 5, May 2013, 329-335.

[41] *Id.*

[42] *Id.*

[43] *Id.*

[44] *Id.*

[45] Sawyer, K. et al, Depression, *Hippocampal Volume Changes, and Cognitive Decline in a Clinical Sample of Older Depressed Outpatients and Non-Depressed Controls*, Aging Mental Health. (2012); 16(6): 753–762.

[46] *Id.*

[47] Diniz, *supra* note 40. Judith Graham, *supra* note 39. Andrea Petersen, *New Therapies Help Patients with Dementia Cope with Depression*, N.Y. Times, Dec. 8, 2019.

[48] *Id.*

[49] Sandee Lamotte, *Poor Sleep Linked to Dangerous Buildup of Plaques Throughout the Body*, CNN.com, Jan.14, 2019.

[50] *Id.*

[51] World Health Organization *supra* note 20. *What's on the Horizon?* Mayo Clinic, https://www.mayoclinic.org/diseases-conditions/alzheimers-disease/in-depth/alzheimers-treatments/art-20047780

[52] *Id.*

[53] *Id.*

[54] *Id.*

[55] Peter Gotsche et al: *Does Long Term Use of Psychiatric Drugs Cause More Harm than Good?* British Medical Journal, May 12, 2015. Sarah Boseley, *Psychiatric Drugs do More Harm than Good, says*

expert, The Guardian, 12 May, 2015.
https://www.theguardian.com/society/2015/may/12/psychiatric-drugs-more-harm-than-good-expert.

[56] *Id.*

[57] Andrea Petersen, *supra* note 39.

[58] Michelle Roberts, *First Drug that Can Slow Alzheimer's Dementia*, BBC, 22 October 2019, https://www.bbc.com/news/health-50137041 *What's on the Horizon?* Mayo Clinic, https://www.mayoclinic.org/diseases-conditions/alzheimers-disease/in-depth/alzheimers-treatments/art-20047780.

[59] Julie Zaugg and Jared Peng, *China Approves Seaweed-based Alzheimer's Drug: It's the First New One in 17 Years,* CNN.com, Nov. 5, 2019. Michelle Roberts, *First Drug that Can Slow Alzheimer's Dementia*, BBC, 22 Oct. 2019.

[60] *Id.*

[61] Choi, H. et. al, *Combined Adult Neurogenesis and BDNF Mimic Exercise Effects on Cognition an Alzheimer's Mouse Model*, Science, Vol. 361 Issue 6406, Sept. 7, 2018. http://science.sciencemag.org/content/361/6406/eaan8821. See, Nagahara, A, and Tuszynski, M., *Potential Therapeutic Uses of BDNF in Neurological and Psychiatric Disorders*, Nature Reviews, Mar. 1, 2011. Blurton-Jones, M. et al. *Neural Stem Cells Improve Cognition via BDNF in Transgenic Model of Alzheimer's Disease*, Proceedings in the National Academy of Sciences 106 (32) Aug. 11, 2009. *BDNF Increases Synaptic Density in Dendrites of Developing Tectal Neurons in Vivo*, Development, 2006, July 133 (13).

[62] *Id.*

[63] Benedict Carey, *To Improve Memory, Tune it Like an Orchestra*, N.Y. Times, Apr. 8, 2019. Benedict Carey, *A Brain Implant Improved Memory, Scientists Report*, Feb. 6, 2018. Ned Herrmann, *What is the Function of the Various Brainwaves*, Scientific American, Dec. 22, 1997. Carl Zimmer, *One Day There May be a Drug to Turbocharge the Brain. Who Should Get it?* Wash. Post April 2, 2019.

[64] Benedict Carey, *A Brain Implant Improved Memory, Scientists Report*, Feb. 6, 2018.

[65] *Id.*

[66] *Id.* Ned Herrmann, *supra* note 63.

[67] Melissa Healy, *Can a Hormone Called Klotho Enhance Cognition and Hold off Dementia, Yes, in Mice at Least*, Wash. Post, Aug. 19, 2017. Zimmer, *supra* note 63. See WHO *supra* note 20.

[68] *Id.*

[69] *Id.*

[70] Erickson et al, *KLOTHO heterozygosity attenuates APOE4-related amyloid burden in preclinical AD*, American Academy of Neurology, Apr. 16, 2019. Aug 13, 2018. Healy, *supra* note 67.

[71] *Id.*

[72] *Id.*

[73] *Id.*

[74] Healy, *supra* note 67. Zimmer supra note 63. WHO *supra* note 20.

[75] Erickson et al, *supra* note 70.

[76] Ji, N. et al, *Aerobic-exercise Stimulated Klotho Upregulation Extends Life Span by Attenuating the Excess Production of Reactive Oxygen Species in the Brain and Kidney*, Experimental and Therapeutic Medicine, Aug. 13, 2018. Matsubara et al; *Aerobic Exercise Training Increases Plasma Klotho Levels and Reduces Arterial Stiffness in Post-Menopausal Women*, AJP Heart and Circulatory Physiology, 306(3) Dec. 2013. Avin, K. et al, *Skeletal Muscle as a Regulator of the Longevity Protein, Klotho, Frontiers in Physiolog*y, 17 June 2014. Healy, *supra* note 67.

[77] Psych Congress Newsroom, *Exploring the Role of GABA in Psychiatric Treatment,* Oct. 3, 2018; Michael J. Breus, *3 Amazing Effects of GABA*, Psychology Today, Jan. 3, 2019. Katherine Ellen Foley, *GABA GABA HEY, The First Drug Specifically for Post-Partum Depression is nearing Approval*, www.qz.com, Aug. 16, 2018. Morgan Kelly, Exercise *Reorganizes the Brain to be More Resilient to Stress*, Princeton University, July 3, 2013.

[78] *Id.*

[79] *Id.*

[80] *Id.*

[81] Abi Millar, *The Drugs Fighting Memory Loss,* www.pharmaceutical-technology.com, 8 Oct. 2019. WUSTL, Neuroscience News, *CRISPR Helps Target Mood Boosting Receptors in the Brain,* neurosciencenews.com. *This is Your Brain on Exercise*, Science Daily, Feb. 25, 2016.

[82] *Id.*

[83] WHO, *supra* note 20. James Gallagher, *Dementia: The Greatest Health Challenge of our Time*, BBC, May 2, 2019.

[84] NAMI, *Mental Health by the Numbers*, https://www.nami.org/Learn-More/Mental-Health-By-the-Numbers. Quick Facts, Alzheimer's Association, https://www.alz.org/alzheimers-dementia/facts-figures.

[85] *Id.*

[86] Danzon Therapy: *Latinos Waltz to Ward off Alzheimer's*, NBC news, Latino, Feb. 3, 2014, nbcnews.com.

[87] WHO, *supra* note 20. Gallagher, *supra* note 83. Ann Norwich, *We're not Prepared for the Coming Dementia Crisis*, Wash. Post Oct. 26,

2018. *Alzheimer's is a Global Epidemic*,
https://alz.org/global/overview.asp

[88] *Alzheimer's is a Global Epidemic*,
https://alz.org/global/overview.asp. James Gallagher, *supra* note 83.
Ann Norwich supra note 87.

[89] Cooper, C. et al. *Modifiable Predictors of Dementia in Mild
Cognitive Impairment: A Systematic Review and Meta-
Analysis. American Journal of Psychiatry*, 2015; Cleveland Clinic,
Mild Cognitive Impairment,
https://my.clevelandclinic.org/health/diseases/17990-mild-cognitive-
impairment.

[90] *Id.*

[91] *Alzheimer's is a Global Epidemic*, *supra* note 88. Gallagher, *supra*
note 83. Danzon Therapy, *supra* note 86. Babula, G.M, *Perspectives on
Ethnic and Racial disparities in Alzheimer's Disease and related
Dementias: Update and Areas of Immediate Need*, Alzheimer's &
Dementia, Journal of the Alzheimer's Association, Feb. 2019, 15(2),
292-312. WHO, *supra* note 20.

[92] *Alzheimer's is a Global Epidemic*, *supra* note 88. WHO, *supra* note
20. Gallagher, *supra* note 83. Danzon Therapy, *supra* note 86.

[93] Ryan Jaslow, *Dementia Costs U.S. Up to $215 billion per year, Study
Finds*, cbsnews.com. April 3, 2013.

[94] WHO, *supra* note 20.

[95] *Id.* WHO, supra note 20. Ryan Jaslow, *supra* note 93. __

[96] *Alzheimer's is a Global Epidemic*, supra note 88. WHO *supra* note
20.

[97] WHO, *supra* note 20.

[98] Maggie Mah, *Positively Determined, Barbara Kalt Wraps Up a
Memorable Career but She is Still on a Mission*." The Almanac, June
29, 2019, https://www.almanacnews.com/news/2019/06/29/positively-
determined

[99] *Id.*

[100] *Id.*

[101] Gallagher, *supra* note 83.

[102] WHO, *supra* note 20.

[103] *Id.*

[104] *Id.*

[105] *Id.* Rachel Dolhum, *Ask the MD: What Is Orthostatic Hypotension?*
The Michael J. Fox Foundation, Foxfeed Blog, Jan. 22, 2015. The
Michael J. Fox Foundation, *Answering Questions on Alzheimer's,
Parkinson's and Dementia*, May 28, 2014,
https://www.michaeljfox.org/news/answering-questions-alzheimers-
parkinsons-and-dementia

[106] *Id.* Pandya M. et al. *Parkinson's Disease: Not Just a Movement Disorder*, Cleveland Clinic Journal of Medicine, Dec. (2008) 75 (12):856-864.

[107] *Id.*

[108] Michelle Ciucci, *Swallowing and Parkinson's Disease*, Michael J. Fox Foundation, Foxfeed Blog, Nov. 5, 2013.

[109] WHO, *supra* note 20.

[110] Heiberger L., et al, *Impact of a Weekly Dance Class on the Functional Mobility and on the Quality of Life of Individuals with Parkinson's Disease*, Frontiers of Aging in Neuroscience, Oct. 10, 2011.

[111] WHO, supra note 20. NIH *Fact Sheets, Parkinson's Disease*, https://www.report.nih.gov/NIHfactsheets/ViewFactSheet.aspx?csid=1 09

[112] The Michael J. Fox Foundation, *Answering Questions on Alzheimer's, supra* note 105.

[113] *Id.*

[114] WHO, *supra* note 20.

[115] Jessie Szalay, *What are Free Radicals?* Live Science, May 2016, https://www.livescience.com/54901-free-radicals.html.

[116] Meredith Gordon Resnick, *I Face a Known Risk from Cancer and an Undetermined Risk from the Scan Used to Detect it. Which is Worse?* Wash. Post. June 8, 2019, https://www.washingtonpost.com/health/i-face-a-known-risk-from-cancer-and-an-undetermined-risk-from-the-scan-used-to-detect-it-which-is-worse/2019/06/07/6f2ed2d8-685e-11e9-82ba-fcfeff232e8f_story.html. Lindsey Bever, *Chuck Norris claims his wife was poisoned during MRI scans, sues for $10 million*, Wash. Post Nov. 8, 2017.

[117] WHO, *supra* note 20.

[118] The Michael J. Fox Foundation, *Answering Questions on Alzheimer's, supra* note 105. *See supra*, note 105.

[119] *Id.*

[120] WHO, *supra* note 20.

[121] *Id.*

[122] *Id.*

[123] *Id.*

[124] *Id. NIH Fact Sheets, supra* note 111.

[125] *Id.*

[126] *Id.*

[127] *Id.*

[128] *Id.*

Chapter II

[1] Ruth A. Richter, A New Rhythm, Dance Benefits Parkinson's Patients, Stanford Medicine, Winter 2017, http://stanmed.stanford.edu/2017winter/dance-for-parkinsons-disease-at-the-stanford-neuroscience-health-center.html

[2] *Id.*

[3] *Id.*

[4] The following sources informed definition of dance: Richard Kraus, Sarah Chapman, *History of the Dance in Art and Education*, Prentice Hall (1981), pp. 5, 12. Lihs, Harriet, *Appreciating dance*, Princeton Dance Company, (2009), p. 2. Walter Sorell, *The Dance Through the Ages*, Grossett & Dunlap, (1967) p.9. Nora Ambrosio, Learning About Dance, Kendall/Hunt (2003), 3

[5] *Id.*

[6] Kraus, *supra* note 4 at 12, 5. Nora Ambrosio, Learning About Dance,Kendall/Hunt, Dubuque, Iowa 2003, p.3; Lihs, Harriet, *supra* note 4 at 1. Sorell, *supra* note 4 at 9.

[7] Kraus, *supra* note 4, pp. 8-9; 15; Curt Sachs, *World History of the Dance*, WW Norton Company (1965), p.3.

[8] *Id.*

[9] *Id.*

[10] Jamake Hightower, *Dance, Rituals of Experience*, Oxford University Press (1996), p.24

[11] *Id.* Kraus, *supra* note 4 at 8.

[12] *Id.*

[13] *Id.*

[14] *Id.*

[15] Ambrosio, *supra* note 4 at 6, Kraus, *supra* note 4 at 15.

[16] Lihs, *supra* note 4 at 1-2.

[17] Kraus, *supra* note 4 at 5, 12. Walter Sorell, *supra* note 4 at 9. Nora Ambrosio, *supra* note 4 at 3. Lihs, *supra* note 4 at 1.

[18] Scott Edwards, *Dancing and the Brain*, The Harvard Mahoney Neuroscience Institute Newsletter. http://neuro.hms.harvard.edu/harvard-mahoney-neuroscience-institute/brain-newsletter/and-brain-series/dancing-and-brain.

[19] British Science Association, Award Lecture, *Getting in the Neural Groove*, Sept. 8, 2017, www.britishsciencefestival.org. Joel Shurkin, *Can Animals Keep a beat?* Inside Science, Feb. 26, 2014.

[20] Ivar Hagendoorn, *The Dancing Brain*, Cerebrum: The Dana Forum on Brain Science, Vol. 5. No. 2, Spring 2003, http://www.ivarhagendoorn.com/files/articles/Hagendoorn-Cerebrum-03.pdf. *Id.*

[21] NIH Fact Sheets, W*hat is Brain Health?* https://brainhealth.nia.nih.gov/.

[22] Jahnavi Sarma, *World Brain Day 2020: 5 habits that Can Damage the Brain*, Healthsite, July 23, 2020.

[23] Hildreth K. el al, *Obesity, Insulin Resistance and Alzheimer's Disease*, Obesity (Silver Spring), Aug. 2012.

[24] Diniz, B.S, et al, *Late-life Depression and Risk of Vascular Dementia and Alzheimer's disease: Systematic review and Meta-analysis of Community-based Cohort Studies*, British J. of Psychiatry, vol. 202, no. 5, May 2013, 329-335. See also, Olga Khazan, *The Startling Link Between Sugar and Alzheimer's*, The Atlantic, Jan. 26, 2018. Zheng, F. et al, HbA1c, *Diabetes and Cognitive Decline: The English Longitudinal Study of Ageing*, Diabetologia, (2018) 61. Harvard Mahoney Neuroscience Institute, *Sugar and the Brain*, https://neuro.hms.harvard.edu/harvard-mahoney-neuroscience-institute/brain-newsletter/and-brain/sugar-and-brain

[25] Martha Graham, *"An Athlete of God,"* NPR Special Series, Historical Archives, Jan. 4, 2006, https://www.npr.org/templates/story/story.php?storyId=5065006

[26] Laland, K. et al, *The Evolution of Dance,* Current Biology, Vol. 26, Issue 1, 11 Jan. 2016, pp. R5-R9. http://www.sciencedirect.com/science/article/pii/S0960982215014256.

[27] Charles Q. Choi, *Early Human 'Lucy' Swung From Trees*, Live Science, Oct. 25, 2012; Michael Mosley, *Why Is There Only One Human Species?* http://www.bbc.com/news/science-environment-13874671. 23 June 2011
What Does it Mean to be Human? Human Characteristics: Brains, Smithsonian.com. http://humanorigins.si.edu/human-characteristics/brains. Jonathan Amos, *African Fossils Put New Spin on Human Origins Story*, http://www.bbc.com/news/science-environment-14824435, Sept. 8, 2011. Pallab Ghoosh, *First Human' Discovered in Ethiopia*, http://www.bbc.com/news/science-environment-31718336. Kevin Loria, *A newly discovered baby skull reveals what the common ancestor of humans and apes may have looked like*, The Business Insider, http://www.businessinsider.com/n-alesi-skull-fossil-discovery-ancestors-apes-humans-kenya-2017-8.

[28] Adam P. Van Arsdale, *Homo Erectus – A Bigger, Smarter, Faster Hominin Lineage*, Nature Education 4 (1): 2013. John Noble Wilford, *When Humans Became Human*, N.Y. Times, Feb. 26, 2002; John Noble Wilford, *Artifacts Revive Debate on Transformation of Human Behavio*r, N.Y. Times, July, 30, 2012; Carl Zimmer, *A Single Migration from Africa Populated the World, Studies Find*, N.Y. Times, Sept. 21, 2016.

[29] *Id.*

[30] Van Arsdale, *supra* note 28.

[31] Wilford, *supra* note 28. Zimmer, *supra* note 28. Smithsonian.com *supra* note 27. *Earliest Humans Not So Different From Us, Research Suggests*, Science daily, Feb. 15, 2011. Aug. 9, 2017. Nathan H. Lents, *Did Neanderthals Speak?* Feb. 9, 2015, https://thehumanevolutionblog.com/2015/02/09/did-neanderthals-speak/.

[32] James Randerson, *How Many Neurons Make a Human Brain,* The Guardian, Feb. 28, 2012. *Brain Facts that Make you Go, "Hmmmmm"* https://faculty.washington.edu/chudler/ffacts.html.

[33] Ferris Jabr, *Know Your Neurons? What is the Ratio of Glia to Neurons in the Brain*, Scientific American, June 13, 2012.

[34] *Id.*

[35] Laland, K. et al, *supra* note 26.

[36] Tia Ghose, *Big Brain Gene Allowed for Evolutionary Expansion of Human Neocortex*, Scientific American, Feb 27, 2015.

[37] Laland K. et al, *supra* note 26.

[38] Scott Edwards, *supra* note 18.

[39] Laland K. et al, *supra* note 26.

[40] Kraus, *supra* note 4 at 14. *Synchrony and exertion during dance independently raise pain threshold and encourage social bonding, Biology Letters,* October 28, 2015. Melissa Hogenboom, *Where Did the Ability to Dance Come From?* bbc.com. Jan. 9, 2017.

[41] Rehfeld, K. et al, *Dancing or Fitness Sport? The Effect of Two Training Programs on Hippocampal Plasticity and Balance Ability*, Frontiers in Human Neuroscience, 2017; 11 DOI: 10.3389/fnhum.2017.00305

[42] Laland K. et al, *supra* note 26.

[43] *Id.*

[44] Scott Edwards, *supra* note 18.

[45] *Id.*

[46] *Id.*

[47] *Id.*

[48] *Id.*

[49] *Id.*

[50] Emily S. Cross, Luca F. Ticini, *Neuroaesthetics and Beyond, New Horizons in Applying the Science of the Brain to the Art of Dance*, www.link.springer.com, Jan. 5, 2011.

[51] Laland K. et al, *supra* note 26. Scott Edwards, *supra* note 18. Tia Ghose, *supra* note 36. Mosley, *supra* note 155. Melissa Hogenboom, *supra* note 40. Christie Aschwanden, *Studies Show the Long-term Positive Effects of Fitness on Cognitive Abilities*, Wash. Post, December 9, 2013.

[52] *See e.g.* Ivar Hagendoorn, *The Dancing Brain*, Cerebrum: The Dana Forum on Brain Science, Vol. 5. No. 2, Spring 2003, http://www.ivarhagendoorn.com/files/articles/Hagendoorn-Cerebrum-03.pdf

[53] Harvard Health Publishing, *Music and Health*, July 2011, https://www.health.harvard.edu/staying-healthy/music-and-health.

[54] *Id.*

[55] *Id.*

[56] Edward Large and Joel Snyder, *Pulse and Meter as Neural Resonance*, The Neurosciences and Music III—Disorders and Plasticity: Ann. N.Y. Acad. Sci. 1169: 46–57 (2009) Oleana Shmahalo, *The Beasts that Keep the Beat*, Quanta Magazine, Mar. 22, 2016.

[57] *Id.*

[58] *Id.*

[59] John Krakauer, *Why Do We Like to Dance and Move to the Beat*, Scientific American, https://www.scientificamerican.com/article/experts-dance/. Jane L. Lee, *Dancing Animals Help Tell Us Why Music Evolved*, National Geographic, Feb. 17, 2014. British Science Association, *supra* note 19.

[60] David J. Linden, *Exercise, Pleasure and the Brain*, Psychology Today, April 21, 2011. Scott Edward, *supra* note 18. Rachel Feltman, *The Sinister Science of Addiction*, Wash. Post, Sept. 14, 2015. Natalie Angier, *Job Description Grows for Our Utility Hormone,* N.Y. Times, May 2, 2011. https://www.nytimes.com/2011/05/03/science/03angier.html.

[61] *Id.*

[62] *Id.*

[63] *Id.*

[64] Krakauer, *supra* note 59.

[65] *Id.* Trisha McNary, *Exercise and its Effects on Serotonin and Dopamine Levels*, https://www.livestrong.com/article/251785-exercise-and-its-effects-on-serotonin-dopamine-levels/.

[66] *Id.*

[67] Jason Daly, *What Happens in the Brain When Music Causes Chills*, Smithsonian.com, June 20, 2016.

[68] Salimpoor V. et al, *The Rewarding Aspects of Music Listening Are Related to Degree of Emotional Arousal*, PLOS One, Oct. 16, 2009. Robert Zatorre and Valarie Salimpoor, *Why Music Makes Our Brains Sing*, N.Y. Times, June 7, 2013. Krakauer, *supra* note 59. *Musical Chills: Why They Give us Thrills*, McGill Newsroom, Jan 10, 2011.

[69] Cross and Ticini, *supra* note 50.

[70] *Id.*

[71] Salimpoor V. et al, *supra* note 68. Robert Zatorre and Valarie Salimpoor, *supra* note 68.

[72] *Id.*

[73] *Id.*

[74] *Id.*

[75] Krakauer, *supra* note 59.

[76] Jason Daly, *supra* note 67.

[77] Don Wade, *Creative Aging Delivers Music as Therapy*, Daily News, Memphis, February 2, 2017.

[78] *Id.*

[79] *Id.*

[80] *Id.*

[81] *Id.*

[82] Trisha McNary, *supra* note 65. David J. Linden, *supra* note 60.

[83] *Id.*

[84] *Id.*

[85] Morgan Kelly, Princeton University, Communications, July 3, *Exercise Reorganizes the Brain to be More Resilient to Stress* 2013. www.princeton.edu. Michael J. Breus, *3 Amazing Effects of GABA*, Psychology Today, Jan. 3, 2019, pschologytoday.com. Psych Congress Newsroom, *Exploring the Role of GABA in Psychiatric Treatment,* Oct. 3, 2018

[86] *Id.*

[87] *Id.*

[88] Michelle Brubaker, *Exercise...It Does a Body Good...20 Minutes Can Act as Anti-Inflammatory*, Jan. 12, 2017, https://health.ucsd.edu/news/releases/Pages/2017-01-12-exercise-can-act-as-anti-inflammatory.aspx.

[89] *Id.*

[90] *Id.*

[91] *Id.*

[92] Exercise *Reorganizes the Brain to be More Resilient to Stress*, Princeton University, July 3, 2013.

[93] *Id. How Does TNF Cause Inflammation*, https://www.webmd.com/rheumatoid-arthritis/how-does-tnf-cause-inflammation#2

[94] *Id.*

[95] *Id.*

[96] Abi Millar, *The Drugs Fighting Memory Loss*, pharmaceutical-technology.com, 8 Oct. 2019. Katherine Ellen Foley, GABA GABA HEY, The First Drug Specifically for Post-Partum Depression is nearing Approval, www.qz.com, Aug. 16, 2018. WUSTL, Neuroscience News, *CRISPR Helps Target Mood Boosting Receptors in the Brain*, neurosciencenews.com.

[97] *This is Your Brain on Exercise*, Science Daily, Feb. 25, 2016, sciencedaily.com. David J. Linden, *supra* note 60.

[98] Christie Aschwanden, *supra* note 51.

[99] *Id. See also,* Blurton-Jones, M. et al. *Neural Stem Cells Improve Cognition via BDNF in Transgenic Model of Alzheimer's Disease*, Proceedings in the National Academy of Sciences (PNAS) https://www.pnas.org/content/106/32/13594; *BDNF Increases Synaptic Density in Dendrites of Developing Tectal Neurons in Vivo*, Development, 2006, Jul. 133 (13) https://www.ncbi.nlm.nih.gov/pubmed/16728478. Aug 11, 2009, 106 (32).

[100] *Id.*

[101] Heidi Godman, *Harvard Health Publishing, Regular Exercise Changes the Brain to Improve Memory and Thinking Skills,* April 9, 2014, https://www.health.harvard.edu/blog/regular-exercise-changes-brain-improve-memory-thinking-skills-201404097110.

[102] *Id.*

[103] *Id.* Kathrin Rehfeld et al, *Dancing or Fitness Sport? supra* note 41.

[104] Christie Aschwanden, *supra* note 51.

[105] *Id.* Yoni Genzer et al, *Effect of Brain Derived neurotropic Factor (BDNF) on Hepatocyte Metabolism*, The International Journal of Biochemistry and Cell Biology, vol 88, July 2017 pp. 69-74.

[106] *Id.*

[107] Melissa Healy, *Can a Hormone Called Klotho Enhance Cognition and Hold off Dementia, Yes, in Mice at Least*, Wash. Post, Aug. 19, 2017.

[108] *Id.*

[109] *Id.*

[110] Matsubara et al; *Aerobic Exercise Training Increases Plasma Klotho Levels and Reduces Arterial Stiffness in Post-Menopausal Women*, AJP Heart and Circulatory Physiology, 306(3) Dec. 2013.

[111] Avin, K. et al, *Skeletal Muscle as a Regulator of the Longevity Protein, Klotho, Frontiers in Physiology*, 17 June 2014.

[112] *Id.*

[113] *Id.*

[114] Gretchen Reynolds, *How Exercise May Keep our Memory Sharp*, N.Y. Times, Jan. 16, 2019, https://www.nytimes.com/2019/01/16/well/move/exercise-brain-memory-irisin-alzheimer-dementia.html.

[115] *Id.*

[116] *Id.*

[117] *Id.*

[118] *Id.*

[119] *Id.*

[120] *Id.*

[121] *Id.*

[122] *Id.* See also, Sisi Wang and Jiyang Pan, *Irisin Ameliorates Depressive-like Behaviors in Rats by Regulating Energy Metabolism, Biochemical and Biophysical Research* Communications, Vol 474, Issue 1, May 20, 2016

[123] Gretchen Reynolds, *Walk, Stretch or Dance? Dancing May Be Best for the Brain*, N.Y. Times, March 29, 2017 https://www.nytimes.com/2017/03/29/well/walk-stretch-or-dance-dancing-may-be-best-for-the-brain.html.

[124] WebMD, *Intelligence May be a Gray and White Matter*, Jan 21, 2005, https://www.webmd.com/brain/news/20050121/intelligence-may-be-gray-white-matter#1.

[125] *Id.*

[126] Reynolds, *Walk, Stretch or Dance? supra* note 123.

[127] *Id.*

[128] *Id.*

[129] *Id.*

[130] *Id.*

[131] Hannah Nichols, *What Happens to the Brain as we Age*, Medical News Today, 29 Aug. 2017, https://www.medicalnewstoday.com/articles/319185.php. Kathleen Phalen, *Steps to a Nimble Mind: Physical and mental Exercise Helps Keep Brain Fit*, American Medical News, Nov. 17, 2000. NIH, *Physical Activity May Reduce Age Related Movement Problems*, https://www.nih.gov/news-events/nih-research-matters/physical-activity-may-reduce-age-related-movement-problems, March 23, 2015.

[132] Robert H. Shmerling, MD, *For People with MS, Can Exercise Change the Brain*, Harvard Health Publishing, Aug. 31, 2017. Feter, N., et al, *Effects of Physical Exercise on Myelin Sheath Regeneration*, Science & Sports, Vol. 33, Issue 1, Feb. 2018, pp. 8- 21.

[133] *Id.*

[134] Isobel Scarisbrick, *Targeting Myelin Metabolism to Enhance Recovery of Function after Spinal Cord Injury*, Neuroregeneration and Neurorehabilitation, Mayo Clinic.

[135] Kathleen Phalen, *supra* note 131.

[136] Bruce Tomaso, *Music Brings Back Memories, Senior dance for Fun and Fitness*, Dallas Morning News, June 1, 2018, https://montanaseniornews.com/music-brings-back-memories-seniors-line-dancing-for-fun-and-fitness/

[137] *Id.*

[138] *Id.*

[139] *Id.*

[140] See *supra* note 131. Hannah Nichols, *supra* note 131

[141] Robert H. Shmerling, MD *supra* note 132. Feter, *supra* note 132

[142] Caroline Ayinon, *Q&A: How Do Dancers Spin without Becoming Dizzy?* Yale-Scientific, Dec. 24, 2013, http://www.yalescientific.org/2013/12/qa-how-do-dancers-spin-without-becoming-dizzy/.

[143] *Id.*

[144] Nigmatullina, Y. et al, *The Neuroanatomical Correlates of Training-Related Perceptuo-Reflex Uncoupling in Dancers*, Cerebral Cortex, vol. Issue 2, 1 Feb. 2015, Pages 554–562.

[145] *Id.*

[146] *Id.*

[147] *Id.*

[148] Ayinon, *supra* note 142.

[149] Gerald Jonas, Dancing, The Pleasure, Power, and Art of Movement, (1998) pp. 31-33.

[150] Alan Burdick, *The Oldest Human Fossil Ever Discovered Have Stories to Tell*, The New Yorker, June 7, 2017. https://www.newyorker.com/tech/elements/the-oldest-human-fossils-ever-discovered-have-stories-to-tell. See Ben Guarino, *Oldest Homo Sapiens Fossil Discovered in Morocco*, Wash. Post, June 7, 2017, https://www.washingtonpost.com/news/speaking-of-science/wp/2017/06/07/oldest-homo-sapiens-fossils-discovered-in-morocco/?utm_term=.94ee4ceb5294.

[151] World Heritage Sites – Rock Shelters of Bhimbetka, , www.asi.nic.in/asi_monu_whs_rockart_bhimbetka_detail.asp.

[152] *Id.*

[153] Joseph Campbell, Primitive Mythology, The Masks of God, Arkana, (1991) p.66, Sachs, *supra* note 7 at 207, 212; Kraus, *supra* note 4 at 31; Ambrosio, *supra* note 4 at 4-5 See also, Archaeology News Network, *Modern Humans Occupied Mas d'Azil Cave 35,000 Years Ago*, https://archaeologynewsnetwork.blogspot.com/2015/06/modern-

humans-occupied-mas-dazil-cave.html#f7fTRwB6y9qxTeKW.99. June
1, 2015; Joshua Hammer, *Finally, the Beauty of France's Chauvet
Cave Makes its Grand Public Debut*, Smithsonian Magazine, April
2015, https://www.smithsonianmag.com/history/france-chauvet-cave-
makes-grand-debut-180954582/#8o5XBmw5pQlszd1H.99

[154] *Id.*

[155] Sachs, *supra* note 7 at 207, 212; Kraus, *supra* note 4 at 31;
Ambrosio, *supra* note 4 at 4-5.

[156] Jo Marcant, *A Journey to the Oldest Cave Paintings in the World,
the discovery in remote part of Indonesia has scholars rethinking the
origins of art – and of humanity*, Smithsonianmag.com, January 2016

[157] *Id.*

[158] *Id.*

[159] John Noble Wilford, *In African Cave, Signs of Ancient Paint
Factory*, N.Y. Times, Oct. 13, 2011. Jo Marcant, *supra* note 156. John
Noble Wilford, *Cave Paintings in Indonesia May Be Among the Oldest
Known*, Oct. 8, 2014.

[160] John Noble Wilford, *When Humans Became Human*, N.Y. Times,
Feb. 26, 2002.

[161] Monte Morin, Neanderthals Smarter than we Thought? LA Times,
May 1, 2014.http://www.latimes.com/science/sciencenow/la-sci-sn-
neanderthals-smarter-than-we-think-20140501-story.html..

[162] *Id.*

[163] Ashley Strickland, *New Findings paint Picture of Neanderthals as
Artists*, CNN Health, Feb. 26, 2018,
https://www.cnn.com/2018/02/22/health/neanderthal-art-symbols-
cognition-study/index.html. Steven Mithen, The Singing Neanderthals,
The Origins of Music, Language, Mind, and Body, Harvard University
Press, 2007.

[164] *Id.*

[165] Micahel Slezak, *Thoroughly Modern Humans Interbred with
Neanderthals*, New Scientist, 22 Oct. 2014,
https://www.newscientist.com/article/dn26435-thoroughly-modern-
humans-interbred-with-neanderthals/. H.G. Orpanides, *DNA Analysis
Reveals How Humans Interbred with Neanderthals*, Wired, 18 Mar
2016, https://www.wired.co.uk/article/dna-analysis-humans-
neanderthals-breeding

[166] Melissa Hogenboom, *supra* note 40.

[167] Amina Khan, *Dance of the Dinosaurs? Strange Gouges Hint at
Bird-like Mating Rituals*, LA Times, No. 17, 2017.
http://www.latimes.com/science/sciencenow/la-sci-sn-dinosaurs-
mating-courtship-birds-20160107-story.html..

[168] *Id..*

[169] *Id.*

[170] Sachs, *supra* note 7 at 176-177.

[171] *Id.*

[172] *Id.*

[173] *Id.*

[174] *Id.*

[175] Anna Newby, *Why Do Animals Dance*? Slate.com Feb. 18 2014.

[176] *Id.*

[177] *Id.*

[178] *Id.*

[179] Oleana Shmahalo, The Beasts that Keep the Beat, Quanta Magazine, https://www.quantamagazine.org/the-beasts-that-keep-the-beat-20160322/, March 22, 2016.

[180] Anna Newby, *supra* note 175.

[181] *Id.*

[182] *Id.*

[183] *Id.*

[184] *Id.*

[185] Melissa Hogenboom, *supra* note 40.

[186] Robert Krulwich, "The List of Animals Who can Truly, Really Dance is Very Short, Who's on It>" www.npr.org. April 1, 2014; Melissa Hogenboom, *supra* note 40. Robert Krulwich, *"The List of Animals Who can Truly, Really Dance is Very Short, Who's on It?"* www.npr.org. April 1, 2014.

[187] *Ten Dazzling Dancers of the Animal Kingdom*, http://www.bbc.com/earth/story/20150626-animal-dancers-that-dazzle. 26 June 2015

[188] *Id.*

[189] *Id.*

[190] *Id.*

[191] *Id.*

[192] *Id.*

[193] Melissa Hogenboom, *supra* note 40.

[194] *Id.*

[195] Kelly-Ann Mills, *Incredible MRI Scan Shows Baby Kicking, Smiling and Dancing in the Womb Thanks to Revolutionary New Technology*, Mirror, 9 Feb. 2017, www.mirror.co.uk *Newborn Infants Detect the Beat in Music*, http://www.musiccognition.nl/newborns/- www.mcg.uva.ni. Melissa Hogenboom, *supra* note 40.

[196] *Id.*

[197] Jane J. Lee, *Dancing Animals Help Tell Us Why Music Evolved*, National Geographic, www.news.nationalgeographic.com, Feb. 14, 2014

[198] *Id.* Kelly-Ann Mills, *supra* note 195.

[199] *Id.*

[200] John Roach, *Babies Use Rhythms to Adapt to their Culture*, National Geographic News, Sept. 21, 2005, www.news.nationalgeographic.com.

[201] *Id.*

[202] *Id.*

[203] Jane J. Lee, *supra* note 197. Kelly-Ann Mills, *supra* note 195.

[204] Marcel Zentner and Tuomas Eerola, *Rhythmic Engagement with Music in Infancy,* Proceedings of the National Academy of Sciences of the United States of America, pnas.org. Vol. 107, no. 13, Feb. 10, 2010. *Babies Are Born to Dance*, Live Science, https://www.livescience.com/6228-babies-born-dance.html. March 15, 2010.
Seriously Science, *Science Proves Babies Love Dancing to Backstreet Boys*, May 21, 2014, www.blogs.discovermagazine.com.

[205] *Id.*

[206] *Id.*

[207] Fuji S. et al., *Precursors of Dancing and Singing to Music in Three-to-Four-Months-Old Infants*, www.ncbi.nlm.nih.gov. May 16, 2014

[208] *Id.*

[209] Hannon, E. et al, *Babies Know Bad Dancing When they See it: Older babies But Not Younger Infants Discriminate between Synchronous and Asynchronous Audiovisual Musical Displays*, Journal of Experimental Child Psychology 159, pp. 159-174 (2017).

[210] Marcel Zentner and Tuomas Eerola *supra* note 204. Live Science, *supra* note 204. Seriously Science, *supra* note 204. Fuji S. et al., *supra* note 207. Hannon, E. et al, *supra* note 209. John Roach, *supra* note 200. Kelly-Ann Mills, *supra* note 195. *Newborn Infants Detect the Beat in Music*, http://www.musiccognition.nl/newborns/- www.mcg.uva.ni. Caspar Addyman, *Scientists Came Up with a Song to Make Babies Happy and Content*, Newsweek.com, Feb 6, 2017.

[211] Kelly-Ann Mills, *supra* note 195. Melissa Hogenboom, *supra* note 40. *Newborn Infants Detect the Beat in Music*, http://www.musiccognition.nl/newborns/- www.mcg.uva.ni.

[212] BBC Radio 3, The Listening Service: *Why Do Babies Love Music So Much?* https://www.bbc.co.uk/programmes/articles/3mrRxx8pbF4Q2hVcSPw2JFj/why-do-babies-love-music-so-much

[213] *Id.*

[214] *Id.*

[215] *Id.*

[216] Kelly-Ann Mills, *supra* note 195.

[217] *Id.*

[218] Caspar Addyman, *supra* note 210.

[219] *'To relieve stress, opt for dance therapy,'* The Pioneer, India, Jan 17, 2011.

[220] *See generally,* Daniel Lieberman, *Is Exercise Really Medicine? An Evolutionary Perspective,"* in Current Sports Medicine Reports 313-319 (2015), https://scholar.harvard.edu/files/dlieberman/files/2015c.pdf.

[221] *Id.* Kelly-Ann Mills, *supra* note 195. Melissa Hogenboom, *supra* note 40.

[222] Science Daily, *"Are Dancers Genetically Different than the Rest of Us? Yes, Says Hebrew University Researcher,"* Science News, Feb. 16, 2006, https://www.sciencedaily.com/releases/2006/02/060213183707.htm.

[223] *Id.*

[224] *Id.*

[225] *Id.*

[226] Carl Zimmer, *Baffling 400,000-Year-Old Clue to Human Origins*, N.Y. Times, Dec. 4, 2013. https://www.nytimes.com/2013/12/05/science/at-400000-years-oldest-human-dna-yet-found-raises-new-mysteries.html

[227] Melissa Hogenboom, *supra* note 40.

[228] Laland, K. et al, *supra* note 26.

[229] *Id.*

[230] *Biology Letters, supra* note 40. Kraus, *supra* note 4, at 14

[231] *Id.*

[232] Steven Mithen, The Singing Neanderthals, The Origins of Music, Language, Mind, and Body, Harvard University Press, 2007.

[233] Mary P. Pflum and Lee Ferran, *Dementia Patients Party Through the Night, New Alzheimer's therapy program gives restless minds room to roam.* ABC news, online, Aug. 4, 2009.

[234] *Id.*

[235] *Id.*

[236] *Id.*

[237] *Id.*

[238] *Id.*

[239] *Id.*

Chapter III

[1] *Dancing to Remember*, University of Washington Brain and Wellness Center, Sept. 5, 2017
http://depts.washington.edu/mbwc/news/article/dancing-to-remember
[2] *Id.*
[3] *Id.*
[4] *Id.*
[5] *Id.*
[6] *Id.*
[7] *Id.*
[8] Verghese, J. et al, *Leisure Activities and the Risk of Dementia in the Elderly*, The New England Journal of Medicine; 2003; 348: 2508-16.
[9] *Id.*
[10] *Id.*
[11] *Id.*
[12] Eckmann and Donald Burke, *Effects of YogaFit vs. Zumba Gold on Cognitive Functioning in an Elderly Female Population,* World Journal of Yoga Physical Therapy and Rehabilitation, Sept. 24, 2014. Barney Calman, *From Parkinson's to Autism, Is there Anything Zumba Can't Tackle?* Daily Mail (online), Oct. 5, 2013. Donna Olmstead, *Studies Show Emotional, Mental and Physical Benefits of Dance*, Albuquerque Journal, Aug. 11, 2014.
[13] Eckmann and Donald Burke, *Effects of YogaFit vs. Zumba Gold on Cognitive Functioning in an Elderly Female Population,* World Journal of Yoga Physical Therapy and Rehabilitation, Sept. 24, 2014. Barney Calman, *From Parkinson's to Autism, Is there Anything Zumba Can't Tackle?* Daily Mail (online), Oct. 5, 2013. Donna Olmstead, *Studies Show Emotional, Mental and Physical Benefits of Dance*, Albuquerque Journal, Aug. 11, 2014.
[14] Eckmann and Donald Burke, *Effects of YogaFit vs. Zumba Gold on Cognitive Functioning in an Elderly Female Population,* World Journal of Yoga Physical Therapy and Rehabilitation, Sept. 24, 2014. Barney Calman, *From Parkinson's to Autism, Is there Anything Zumba Can't Tackle?* Daily Mail (online), Oct. 5, 2013. Donna Olmstead, *Studies*

Show Emotional, Mental and Physical Benefits of Dance, Albuquerque Journal, Aug. 11, 2014.

[15] *Id.*

[16] Donna Olmstead, *supra* note 12.

[17] Lenny Bernstein, *More Evidence that Exercise Can Help Fight Alzheimer's Disease*, Wash. Post, Dec. 16, 2014. CDC, *Dance Your Way to Better Brain Health*, https://www.cdc.gov/features/alzheimers-and-exercise/index.html.

[18] *Id.*

[19] *Id.*

[20] Trish Vella-Burrows and Lian Wilson, *Remember to Dance, Evaluating the impact of dance activities for people in different stages of dementia*, Sidney De Haan Research Centre for Arts and Health, p. 12, https://www.greencandledance.com/wp-content/uploads/2014/02/141-KC-15-SDH_DanceDementia_Report-2016-proof-08.pdf

[21] *See generally*, Scott Edwards, *Dancing and the Brain*, The Harvard Mahoney Neuroscience Institute Newsletter. http://neuro.hms.harvard.edu/harvard-mahoney-neuroscience-institute/brain-newsletter/and-brain-series/dancing-and-brain.

[22] Rehfeld, K. et al, *Dancing or Fitness Sport? The Effect of Two Training Programs on Hippocampal Plasticity and Balance Ability*, Frontiers in Human Neuroscience, 2017; 11 DOI: 10.3389/fnhum.2017.00305

[23] *Id.*

[24] *Id.*

[25] *Id.*

[26] *Id.*

[27] *Id.*

[28] *Id.*

[29] *Id.*

[30] *Id.*

[31] *Id.*

[32] *Id.*

[33] *Id.*

[34] *Id.*

[35] Rehfeld, K, et al. *Dance Training is Superior to Repetitive Physical Exercise in Inducing Brain Plasticity in the Elderly. PLOS one* vol. 13,7. Jul. 11, 2018.

[36] *Id.*

[37] *Id.*

[38] *Id.*

[39] *Id.*

[40] *Id.*

[41] *Id.*

[42] *Id.*

[43] *Id.*

[44] *Id.*

[45] *Id.*

[46] Comment by Alice P. Simpson, in Gretchen Reynolds, *Walk, Stretch or Dance? Dancing May Be Best for the Brain*, N.Y. Times, March 29, 2017. [Comments] https://www.nytimes.com/2017/03/29/well/walk-stretch-or-dance-dancing-may-be-best-for-the-brain.html#commentsContainer.

[47] *Id.*

[48] *Id.*

[49] *Id.*

[50] *Id.*

[51] *Id.*

[52] *Id.*

[53] Comment by VKG, in Gretchen Reynolds, *Walk, Stretch or Dance? supra* note 46

[54] *Id.*

[55] *Id.*

[56] *Id.*

[57] Burzynska, Agnieszka Z et al. *White Matter Integrity Declined Over 6-Months, but Dance Intervention Improved Integrity of the Fornix of Older Adults. Frontiers in Aging Neuroscience* vol. 9 59. Mar. 16, 2017. See also, Gretchen Reynolds, *Walk, Stretch or Dance? supra* note 46.

[58] *Id.*

[59] *Id.*

[60] *Id.*

[61] *Id.*

[62] *Id.*

[63] Comment by William (Santa Barbara) in Gretchen Reynolds, *Walk, Stretch or Dance? supra* note 46.

[64] *Id.*

[65] *Id.*

[66] *Id.*

[67] *Id.*

[68] *Id.*

[69] *Id.*

[70] Comment by Lisa N. (Los Angeles) in Reynolds, *Walk, Stretch or Dance? supra* note 46.

[71] Id.

[72] Eyre, H. et al, *Changes in Neural Connectivity and Memory Following a Yoga Intervention for Older Adults: A Pilot Study*. Journal of Alzheimer's Disease, vol. 52,2 (2016): 673-84. See also, Gretchen Reynolds, Yoga May be Good for the Brain, N.Y. Times, June 1, 2016. https://well.blogs.nytimes.com/2016/06/01/yoga-may-be-good-for-the-brain/

[73] *Id.*

[74] *Id.*

[75] *Id.*

[76] *Id.*

[77] *Id.*

[78] Id.

[79] Id.

[80] Id.

[81] Raji, C. et al. *Longitudinal Relationships between Caloric Expenditure and Gray Matter in the Cardiovascular Health Study*. Journal of Alzheimer's Disease, vol. 52,2 (2016): 719-29. See also, Gretchen Reynolds, *Walk, Stretch or Dance? supra* note 46.

[82] Raji, *supra* note 81.

[83] *Id.*

[84] *Id.*

[85] *Id.*

[86] *Id.*

[87] *Id.*

[88] *Id.*

[89] *Id.*

[90] *Id.*

[91] *Id.*

[92] *Id.*

[93] Lenny Bernstein, *supra* note 17. CDC, *Dance Your Way to Better Brain Health*, *supra* note 17.

[94] *Id.*

[95] Hörder, J. et al, *Midlife Cardiovascular Fitness and Dementia: A 44-year Longitudinal Population Study in Women*. Neurology, Apr. 10, 2018, 90 (15).

[96] *Id.*

[97] *Id.*

[98] *Id.*

[99] *Id.*

[100] *Id.*

[101] Kelly Servick, *How Does Exercise Keep Your Brain Young?* Science Sept. 6, 2018. Alzforum, *44 Year Study Ties Midlife Fitness to*

Lower Dementia Risk, https://www.alzforum.org/news/research-news/44-year-study-ties-midlife-fitness-lower-dementia-risk.

[102] Kovacevic, A. et al, *The Effects of Aerobic Exercise Intensity on Memory in Older Adults*, Journal of Applied Physiology, Nutrition and Metabolism, Oct. 30, 2019; *See also*, Gretchen Reynolds, *The Right Kind of Exercise May Boost Memory and Lower Dementia Risk*, N.Y Times, Nov. 6, 2019, https://www.nytimes.com/2019/11/06/well/move/exercise-dementia-memory-alzheimers-brain-seniors-middle-age.html

[103] *Id.*

[104] *Id.*

[105] *Id.*

[106] *Id.*

[107] *Id.*

[108] *The Right Kind of Exercise May Boost Memory and Lower Dementia Risk*, N.Y Times, Nov. 6, 2019, https://www.nytimes.com/2019/11/06/well/move/exercise-dementia-memory-alzheimers-brain-seniors-middle-age.html.

[109] Tari, A. et al, *Temporal Changes in Cardiovascular Fitness and Risks of Dementia Incidence and Mortality: A Population-based Prospective Cohort Study*, The Lancet Public Health, vol. 4, issue 11, Nov. 1, 2019. *See also*, Gretchen Reynolds, *The Right Kind of Exercise May Boost Memory and Lower Dementia Risk*, N.Y Times, Nov. 6, 2019, https://www.nytimes.com/2019/11/06/well/move/exercise-dementia-memory-alzheimers-brain-seniors-middle-age.html.

[110] *Id.*

[111] *Id.*

[112] *Id.*

[113] Norwegian University of Science and Technology, *Improved Fitness Can Mean Living Longer without Dementia,* Medical Express, Nov. 12, 2019.

[114] McKinley, P. et al, *Argentine Tango dancing Improves Balance and Complex Task Performance in at-Risk Elderly*, Gait & Posture, 21: 1 (June 2005) p.117. McGill Newsroom, *Shall We Dance? Doing the Tango Improves the Aging Brain*, Nov. 23, 2005, https://www.mcgill.ca/newsroom/channels/news/shall-we-dance-17607

[115] McGill Newsroom, *supra* note 114.

[116] *Id.*

[117] McKinley, P. et al, *supra* note 114.

[118] *Id.*

[119] Hackney, M. et al, *Effects of tango on functional mobility in Parkinson's disease: a preliminary study, Journal of Neurologic Physical Therapy*, Vol. 31, Issue 4, pp. 173-179. Dec. 12, 2007

[120] *Id.*

[121] *Id.*

[122] Heiberger L. et al, *Impact of a Weekly Dance Class on the Functional Mobility and on the Quality of Life of Individuals with Parkinson's Disease*, Frontiers of Aging in Neuroscience, Oct. 10, 2011.

[123] *Id.*

[124] *Id.*

[125] *Id.*

[126] *Id.*

[127] *Id.*

[128] *Id.*

[129] *Id.*

[130] *Id.*

[131] *Id.*

[132] Id.

[133] *Id.*

[134] *Id.*

[135] *Id.*

[136] *Id.*

[137] Id.

[138] *Id.*

[139] *Id.*

[140] *Id.*

[141] *Id.*

[142] *Id.*

[143] *Id.* See also, video of the dance at: http://www.uniklinik-freiburg.de/neurologie/live/forschung/xpeeg.html.

[144] Ryan P. Duncan and Gammon Earhart, *Are the Effects of Community Based Dance on Parkinson's Disease Severity, Balance and Functional Mobility Reduced with Time? A Two-year Prospective Pilot Study*, The Journal of Alternative and Complementary Medicine Vol. 20, No. 10, Oct. 2014.

[145] *Id.*

[146] *Id.*

[147] *Id.*

[148] *Id.*

[149] *Id.*

[150] *Id.*

[151] *Id.* See also, Madeleine E. Hackney and Gammon Earhart, *Effects of Dance on Gait and Balance in Parkinson's Disease: A Comparison of Partnered and Nonpartnered Dance Movement*, vol. 24 issue: 4, pp. 384-392, May 1, 2010. Ryan P. Duncan and Gammon Earhart,

Randomized Control Trial in Community Based Dancing to Modify Disease Progression in Parkinson's Disease, Neurorehabilitation and Neural Repair, vol. 26 issue: 2, page(s): 132-143; Feb. 1, 2012.

[152] Romenets, S. et al, *Tango for treatment of motor and non-motor manifestations in Parkinson's disease: A randomized control study*, Complementary Therapies in Medicine, vol. 23, issue 2, Apr. 2015, Pages 175-184

[153] *Id.*

[154] *Id.*

[155] *Id.*

[156] *Id.*

[157] *Id.*

[158] Washington University School of Medicine, *Dancing to Ease Disease: Tango with a Beneficial Beat*, June 24, 2016. https://neuro.wustl.edu/News/Dancing-To-Ease-Disease-Tango-With-A-Beneficial-Beat

[159] *Id.* See also, Madeleine Hackney, *Adapted Tango: Bringing Artistry to Rehabilitation*, LER Magazine, June 2015 https://lermagazine.com/article/adapted-tango-bringing-artistry-to-rehabilitation

[160] Scott Edwards, *supra* note 21.

[161] *Id.*

[162] *Id.*

[163] Li, F. et al, *Tai Chi and Postural Stability in Patients with Parkinson's Disease*, The New England Journal of Medicine, Feb. 9, 2021, 366:511-519.

[164] *Id.*

[165] *Id.*

[166] *Id.*

[167] *Id.*

[168] *Id.*

[169] *Id.*

[170] *Id.*

[171] Sara Houston and Ashley McGill, *Researching Dance for Parkinson's,* Dance of Parkinson's Project, The University of Roehampton, http://roehamptondance.com/parkinsons/

[172] *Id.*

[173] *English National Ballet's Dance for Parkinson's Program Research Revealed by Roehampton Academics*, University of Roehampton, https://www.roehampton.ac.uk/dance/news/english-national-ballet-dance-for-parkinsons-research-revealed-by-roehampton-academics/

[174] *Id.*

[175] *Id.*

[176] *Id.*

[177] *Id.*

[178] *Id.*

[179] *Id.*

[180] *Id.*

[181] *Id.* See also, Sara Houston and Ashley McGill, *supra* note 171.

[182] Washington University School of Medicine, *supra* note 158. McGill Newsroom, *supra* note 114.

[183] *English National Ballet's Dance for Parkinson's Program Research Revealed by Roehampton Academics*, University of Roehampton, https://www.roehampton.ac.uk/dance/news/english-national-ballet-dance-for-parkinsons-research-revealed-by-roehampton-academics/

[184] Ruth Richter, A New Rhythm, Dance Benefits Parkinson's Patients, Stanford Medicine, Winter 2017, http://stanmed.stanford.edu/2017winter/dance-for-parkinsons-disease-at-the-stanford-neuroscience-health-center.html. *See also*, Westheimer, O. *et al. Dance for PD: a preliminary investigation of effects on motor function and quality of life among persons with Parkinson's disease (PD). J Neural Transmission* 122, 1263–1270 (2015). https://doi.org/10.1007/s00702-015-1380-x

[185] *Id.*

[186] Washington University School of Medicine, *supra* note 158. McGill Newsroom, *supra* note 114.

[187] *Id.*

[188] *Fighting Dementia with Dance Therapy*, The Nation (Thailand), April 2, 2017.

[189] Ruth Richter, *supra* note 184.

[190] *Id.*

[191] *Id.*

[192] Washington University School of Medicine, *supra* note 158.

[193] Ruth Richter, *supra* note 184.

[194] *Id.*

[195] *Id.*

[196] *Id.*

[197] Katie Demeria, *Dancing with Parkinson's Disease,* Richmond Times Dispatch, Nov. 14, 2016.

[198] *Id.*

[199] *Id.*

[200] Ruth Richter, *supra* note 184.

[201] *Id.*

[202] *See generally*, Sarah Hampson, *Getting Their Groove Back; From the gym to the ballroom, personal trainer Sarah Robichaud shows Parkinson's patients like Andy Barrie how the tango and waltz can*

loosen muscles and lift spirits, The Globe and Mail, Mar. 3, 2008; Gloria Hochman, *Dance Classes Help Parkinson's Patients Stay Limber*, The Philadelphia Inquirer, July 16, 2013; Sandra Lorenzo, *For Parkinson's Patients, Dancing the Tango Can Help Reconnect Mind and Body*, Huffington Post, Apr. 17, 2015. Ese Olumhense, *Parkinson's Disease Progression Can be Slowed with Vigorous Exercise Study Shows*, Chicago Tribune, Dec. 11, 2017.

[203] Heiberger L., et al, *Impact of a Weekly Dance Class on the Functional Mobility and on the Quality of Life of Individuals with Parkinson's Disease*, Frontiers of Aging in Neuroscience, Oct. 10, 2011.

[204] Rehfeld, K, et al. *Dance training is superior to repetitive physical exercise in inducing brain plasticity in the elderly. PLOS one* vol. 13,7. Jul. 11, 2018.

[205] *Id.*

[206] *Id.*

[207] Ruth Richter, *supra* note 184.

[208] *Id.*

[209] *Id.*

[210] Verghese, *supra* note 8. Scott Edwards, *supra* note 21.

[211] Heiberger L., et al, *Impact of a Weekly Dance Class on the Functional Mobility and on the Quality of Life of Individuals with Parkinson's Disease*, Frontiers of Aging in Neuroscience, Oct. 10, 2011..

[212] Verghese, *supra* note 8. Scott Edwards, *supra* note 21.

[213] Rehfeld, K, et al. *Dance training is superior to repetitive physical exercise in inducing brain plasticity in the elderly. PLOS one* vol. 13,7. Jul. 11, 2018.

[214] John Krakauer, *Why Do We Like to Dance and Move to the Beat*, Scientific American, https://www.scientificamerican.com/article/experts-dance/. Scott Edwards, *supra* note 21.

[215] Heiberger L., et al, *Impact of a Weekly Dance Class on the Functional Mobility and on the Quality of Life of Individuals with Parkinson's Disease*, Frontiers of Aging in Neuroscience, Oct. 10, 2011.

[216] *Id.*

[217] Karen Weintraub, *Is Art Therapy the Answer for Dementia? Making music, painting, or dancing — and seeing or hearing it — may be the most effective treatment for dementia to date*, The Boston Globe, Nov. 27, 2012. Heiberger, L. *supra* note 215. Scott Edwards, *supra* note 21.

[218] *Id.*

[219] See generally, Rehfeld, K. et al, *Dancing or Fitness Sport? The Effect of Two Training Programs on Hippocampal Plasticity and Balance Ability*, Frontiers in Human Neuroscience, 2017; 11 DOI: 10.3389/fnhum.2017.00305. Verghese, *supra* note 8. Edwards, *supra* note 21.

[220] Comment by Lisa, in Gretchen Reynolds, *Walk, Stretch or Dance? supra* note 46.

[221] *Id.*

[222] *Id.*

[223] *Id.*

[224] *Id.*

[225] Rehfeld, K, et al. *Dance training is superior to repetitive physical exercise in inducing brain plasticity in the elderly. PLOS one* vol. 13,7. Jul. 11, 2018. Jonathan Grinstein, *How Exercise Might 'Clean' the Alzheimer's Brain, Hints at Potential Treatments for Age-Related memory Loss*, Scientific American, Oct. 16, 2018, https://www.scientificamerican.com/article/how-exercise-might-clean-the-alzheimers-brain1/. Choi, H. et. al, *Combined Adult Neurogenesis and BDNF Mimic Exercise Effects on Cognition an Alzheimer's Mouse Model*, Science, Vol. 361 Issue 6406, Sept. 7, 2018. http://science.sciencemag.org/content/361/6406/eaan8821. Krakauer, *supra* note 214. Sarah Klein, *This is What Happens to your Body When You Exercise*, HuffPost, Dec. 6, 2017. Reynolds, *Walk, Stretch, or Dance? supra* note 46. Scott Edwards, *supra* note 21. WebMD, *Causes of Alzheimer's Disease*, https://www.webmd.com/alzheimers/guide/alzheimers-causes-risk-factors; Hannah Nichols, *What Happens to the Brain as we Age*, Medical News Today, 29 Aug. 2017, https://www.medicalnewstoday.com/articles/319185.php. Jessica Boddy, *Watching Neurons talk in a Living Brain*, Science, Sciencemag.org, July 21, 2016. Benedict Carey, *Scientists Can Create Speech from Brain Signals*, N.Y. Times, Apr. 24, 2019. Howard Hughes medical Institute, *How to 'Read' the Brain Signals Underlying Human Speech*, https://www.hhmi.org/news/how-to-read-the-brain-signals-underlying-human-speech.

[226] *Id.*

[227] Kathleen Phalen, *Steps to a Nimble Mind: Physical and mental Exercise Helps Keep Brain Fit*, American Medical News, Nov. 17, 2000.

[228] Emily S. Cross, Luca F. Ticini, *Neuroaesthetics and Beyond, New Horizons in Applying the Science of the Brain to the Art of Dance*, www.link.springer.com, Jan. 5, 2011.

[229] Phalen, *supra* note 227.

[230] *Id.*

[231] Rehfeld, K, et al. *Dance training is superior to repetitive physical exercise in inducing brain plasticity in the elderly*. *PLOS one* vol. 13,7. Jul. 11, 2018 Jonathan Grinstein, *How Exercise Might 'Clean' the Alzheimer's Brain, Hints at Potential Treatments for Age-Related memory Loss*, Scientific American, Oct. 16, 2018, https://www.scientificamerican.com/article/how-exercise-might-clean-the-alzheimers-brain1/. Richard Powers, *Use it or Lose it, Dancing Makes You Smarter, Longer*, Stanford Dance, https://socialdance.stanford.edu/syllabi/smarter.htm

[232] Powers, *supra* note 231. Verghese, *supra* note 8.

[233] Ruth Richter, *supra* note 184.

[234] Verghese, *supra* note 8.

[235] Hampson, *supra* note 202.

[236] *Id.*

[237] Harry Kerasidis, *Rebuilding the Brain from Concussions*, Psychology Today, Mar. 24, 2017.

[238] Sara Houston *(Investigative Study 2) supra* note 171.

[239] *Id.*

[240] *Id.*

[241] Verghese, *supra* note 8. Debra Goldschimdt, *Is Alzheimer's Preventable?* https://www.cnn.com/2015/06/23/health/alzheimers-early-intervention/index.html. June 19, 2018. See also, Styliani Douka et al, *Greek Traditional Dances: A Way to Support Intellectual, Psychological, and Motor Functions in Senior Citizens at Risk of Neurodegeneration*, Frontiers in Aging Neuroscience., 25 Jan. 2019

[242] Powers, *supra* note 231.

[243] *Id.*

[244] Dan Schawbel, *Dr. Daniel Amen: How to Use Your Brain to be a More Effective Worker*, Forbes, Dec. 4, 2017.;

[245] Trish Vella-Burrows and Lian Wilson, *supra* note 20.

[246] Phalen, *supra* note 227.

[247] Debra Goldschimdt, *supra* note 241.

Chapter IV

[1] Richard Kraus, Sarah Chapman, *History of the Dance in Art and Education*, Prentice Hall (1981), p. 11. Harriet Lihs, *Appreciating dance*, Princeton Dance Company, (2009), p. 5

[2] Lucian "On the Dance," quoted in Maria-Gabrielle Wosien, Sacred Dance, Encounter with the Gods, p.7, Thames and Hudson, New York (1986), p.8.

[3] Isabella Pericleous, *Healing Through Movement: Dance/Movement Therapy for major Depression*, Senior Seminar in Dance 2011, (Director: Professor L. Gafarola) Columbia University.

[4] Kraus, *supra* note 1, 31-32.

[5] *Id.*

[6] *Id.*

[7] Curt Sachs, World History of the Dance, WW Norton Company, Inc. NY, (1965), pp. 29. Nora Ambrosio, Learning About Dance,Kendall/Hunt, Dubuque, Iowa 2003, 4-5.

[8] Egyptian Art and Architecture, Relief Sculpture and Painting, https://www.britannica.com/art/Egyptian-art/Relief-sculpture-and-painting

[9] Sachs, *supra* note 7 at 86-87.

[10] Walter Sorell, *The Dance Through the Ages*, Grossett & Dunlap, (1967), p. 26

[11] Joshua Mark, Isis, Ancient History Encyclopedia, February 19, 2016, https://www.ancient.eu/isis/.

[12] *Id.*

[13] Kraus, *supra* note 1 at 32-33. Ricky Weiss, *Music Therapy*, Wash. Post, July 5, 1994

[14] Kraus, *supra* note 1 at 31-33, 37; Sorell, *supra* note 10 at 21-22, 32.

[15] Sorell, *supra* note 10 at 22.

[16] *Id.*

[17] Sorell, *supra* note 10 at 27. *See generally,* Irena Lexova, Ancient Egyptian Dances, Dover, NY (2000). *See also,* Irena Lexova , History of Dance in Egypt, https://sites.google.com/site/danceinegypt/sources/books/ancient-egyptian-dances.

[18] Sachs, *supra* note 7 at 221. Sorell, *supra* note 10 at 26

[19] Sachs, *supra* note 7, p. 145. Maria-Gabrielle Wosien, *supra* note 2 at 7.

[20] *Id.*

[21] *Id.*

[22] Ben-Ami Scharfstein, Art Without Borders, University of Chicago, (2009), p. 122. Wosien, *supra* note 2 at 7-8.

[23] *Id.*

[24] *Id.* Nataraja, Hindu Mythology, https://www.britannica.com/topic/Shiva

[25] Thematic Guide to World Mythology.doc wolfweb.unr.edu/... Phyllis Jestice, Holy People of the World, A Cross-Cultural Encyclopedia, (2004) p. 665

[26] Thematic Guide to World Mythology.doc wolfweb.unr.edu/...

[27] Mildred Boyd, Dancing for the Gods, http://www.chapala.com/chapala/magnifecentmexico/dancinggods/dancinggods.html. www.worldartswest.org/main/discipline.asp?i=49;

[28] *Id.*

[29] *Id.*

[30] *Id.*

[31] Sachs, *supra* note 7 at 90.

[32] *Id.*

[33] *Id.*

[34] Sydney Carter, Lord of the Dance, https://genius.com/Sydney-carter-lord-of-the-dance-lyricsThe Jesus Question, https://thejesusquestion.org/2012/02/13/jesus-the-dancer-part-1-sydney-carters-lord-of-the-dance/. Sydney Carter's song was (adapted from the Shaker song "Simple Gifts" by Joseph Brackett)

[35] Eurynome Greek creation myth www.paleothea.com/Myths/Eurynome.html. See also, Robert Graves, The Greek Myths, Penguin, 1st ed. (1955); Sachs, 90.

[36] *Id.*

[37] *Id.*

[38] Sorell, supra note 10 at 22.

[39] Marcelo Gleiser, The Dancing Universe, From Creation Myths to the Big Bang, 32-33. Dartmouth College Press, Hanover, New Hampshire, (1997), pp. 31-33, 41.

[40] Id.

[41] *Id.*

[42] Ziauddin Sardar, *Pythagoras by Kitty Ferguson*, Independent, Oct. 8, 2010, https://www.independent.co.uk/arts-entertainment/books/reviews/pythagoras-by-kitty-ferguson-2100696.html

[43] Marcelo Gleiser, *supra* note 39 at 32-33

[44] *Id.*

[45] Lucian "On the Dance" supra note 2.

[46] *Id.*

[47] Sachs, *supra* note 7 at 131, *See also*, Sachs, *supra* note 7 at 148-149. Sorell, *supra* note 10 at 22.
[48] Marcelo Gleiser, supra note 39 at 32-33
[49] Wosien, *supra* note 2 at 8, Sorell, *supra* note 10 at 52
[50] Kraus, *supra* note 1 at 37; Sorell, *supra* note 10 at 22, 32; Sachs, *supra* note 7 at 242.
[51] Sachs, *supra* note 7 at 242, Sorell, *supra* note 10 at 32.
[52] Kraus, *supra* note 1 at 41.
[53] *Id.*
[54] Sorell, *supra* note 10 at 30
[55] *Id.*
[56] Jamake Hightower, *Dance, Rituals of Experience*, Oxford University Press (1996), p.42.
[57] Sorell, *supra* note 10 at 27
[58] Sachs, *supra* note 7 at 239-240.
[59] Shashi Agarwal, *Cardiovascular Benefits of Exercise,* International Journal of General Medicine, 5: 541–545. (2012) doi: 10.2147/IJGM.S30113
[60] Ricky Weiss, *supra* note 13.
[61] Shashi Agarwal, *supra* note 59.
[62] *Id.*
[63] Sachs, *supra* note 7 at 239-240
[64] *Id.*
[65] *Id.*
[66] Sorell, *supra* note 10 at 27
[67] Sachs, *supra* note 7 at 239. Kraus, *supra* note 1 at 40
[68] Kraus, *supra* note 1 at 39. See also, Gerald Jonas, Dancing, The Pleasure, Power, and Art of Movement, (1998) pp. 40-41
[69] Kraus, *supra* note 1 at 37.
[70] Sachs, *supra* note 7 at 18.
[71] Kraus, supra note 1 at 40.
[72] *Id.* at 109.
[73] *Id.*
[74] *Id.* at 39
[75] *Id.* at 109.
[76] *Id.*
[77] *Id.* at 110
[78] Sorell, *supra* note 10 at 32. Jonas, *supra* note 68 at 41
[79] *Id.*
[80] Sorell, *supra* note 10 at 32. Kraus, *supra* note 1 at 45
[81] *Id.*
[82] Jonas, *supra* note 68 at 41
[83] Kraus, *supra* note 1 at 42-43

[84] Sachs, *supra* note 7 at 249. Jonas, *supra* note 68 at 116

[85] Anthony Shay, *Dance and Jurisprudence in the Islamic Middle East*, http://thebestofhabibi.com/vol-19-no2-sept-2002/dance-and-jurisprudence/

[86] Sorell, *supra* note 10 at 35. Kraus, *supra* note 1 at 46

[87] Kraus, *supra* note 1 at 43.

[88] *Id.* at 43 – 44.

[89] Sorell, *supra* note 10 at 35. Kraus, *supra* note 1 at 43-44.

[90] *Id.*

[91] Kraus, *supra* note 1 at 42-43.

[92] Sorell, *supra* note 10 at 22.

[93] Lihs, *supra* note 1 at 13.

[94] Sorell *supra* note 10 at 24; Kraus, *supra note 1* at 43.

[95] Highwater, *supra* note 56 at 43-44.

[96] *Id.*

[97] Sorell, *supra* note 10 at 24.

[98] Kraus, *supra* note 1, at 43, 50-52; Sorell, *supra* note 10 at 38

[99] Hightower, *supra* note 56 at 47. *See also*, Jonas, *supra* note 68 at 41-42. Kraus, *supra* note 1 at 43, 52. Sorell, *supra* note 10 at 24, 38.

[100] Sachs, *supra* note 7 at 248-249. Hightower, *supra* note 56 at 47.

[101] Jonas, *supra* note 68 at 42, 47. Kraus, *supra* note 1 at 43, 52. Highwater, *supra* note 56 at 47. Sorell, *supra* note 10 at 24, 38.

[102] Kraus, *supra* note 1 at 52. Jonas, *supra* note 68 at 47. Sorell, *supra* note 10 at 38.

[103] Highwater, *supra* note 56 at 47. Kraus, *supra* note 1 at 43.

[104] Sorell, supra note 10 at 24. Hightower, *supra* note 56 at 47. Kraus, *supra* note 1 at 43.

[105] Sachs, *supra* note 7 at 63.

[106] Kraus, *supra* note 1, at 28

[107] *Id.*

[108] Lihs, *supra* note 1 at 9.

[109] Sachs, *supra* note 7 at 64.

[110] *Id.*

[111] *Id.*

[112] *Id.* at 63.

[113] *Id.* at 54, 28.

[114] Kraus, *supra* note 1 at 11.

[115] Lihs, *supra* note 1 at 5

[116] Angela Shelf Medearis and Micheal R. Medearis, Dance, African American Arts series, Twenty First Century Books (1997), pp. 6-7.

[117] Lihs, *supra* note 1 at 5

[118] Kraus, *supra* note 1 at 11-12, 14. Michel Huett, The Dance, Art, and Ritual of Africa, Pantheon (1978), p. 18

[119] Kraus, *supra* note 1 at 11-12, 14.

[120] *Id.* at 14.

[121] Medearis, supra note 116 at 6-7.

[122] Highwater, *supra* note 56 at 127.

[123] Huett, *supra* note 118 at 18 (Introduction by Jean Laude, Professor of Art History, Paris University 1, Sorbonne).

[124] *Id.*

[125] Kraus, *supra* note 1 at 14.

[126] *Id.*

[127] Sorell, *supra* note 10 at 52-56.

[128] *Id.* at 52.

[129] Lihs, *supra* note 1 at 14. Sachs, *supra* note 7 at 233.

[130] Sachs, *supra* note 7 at 233. Lihs, *supra* note 1 at 14.

[131] Sachs, *supra* note 7, at 233. Sorell, *supra* note 10 at 52.

[132] *Id.*

[133] Sorell, *supra* note 10 at 56.

[134] *Id.* at 53, 56.

[135] *Id.*

[136] *Id.* at 56.

[137] Huett, *supra* note 118 at 16-17.

[138] *Id.*

[139] *Id.* at 17.

[140] *Id.*

[141] *Id.* at 16

[142] *Id.*

[143] *Id.* 16-17; Sachs, *supra* note 7 at 51

[144] Sachs *supra* note 7 at 51.

[145] *Id.* at 50, 52-53.

[146] *Id.* at 50. Sorell, *supra* note 10 at 49, 59.

[147] Sachs, *supra* note 7 at 50.

[148] Kraus, *supra* note 1 at 23.

[149] *Id.*

[150] Sachs, *supra* note 7 at 46-47.

[151] Kraus, *supra* note 1 at 23.

[152] Sachs, *supra* note 7 at 27.

[153] *Id.* at 26-28.

[154] *Id.* at 26, 88.

[155] *Id.* at 88, 28.

[156] Nicole M. Monteiro and Dianna J. Wall, *African Dance as Healing Modality Throughout the Diaspora: The Use of Ritual and Movement to Work Through Trauma*, The Journal of Panafrican Studies, Vol. 4, no. 6, Sept. 2011.

[157] *Id.*

[158] *Id.*

[159] *Id.*

[160] *Id.*

[161] *Id.*

[162] *Id.*

[163] *Id.*

[164] *Id.*

[165] *Id.*

[166] Huett, *supra* note 118 at 30.

[167] *Id.*

[168] Huett, *supra* note 118 at 30. Lihs, *supra* note 1 at 12.

[169] Huett, *supra* note 118 at 30.

[170] *Id.* at 27.

[171] *Id.* at 27-28.

[172] *Id.* at 28.

[173] *Id.*

[174] Lihs, *supra* note 1 at 12.

[175] *Id.*

[176] Huett, *supra* note 118 at 13.

[177] Highwater, *supra* note 56 at 23.

[178] *Id.* at 36.

[179] Huett, *supra* note 118 at 19.

[180] Highwater, *supra* note 56 at 33, 35-36, 40

[181] *Id.* at 35.

[182] Sorell, *supra* note 10 at 50.

[183] Highwater, *supra* note 56 at 27.

[184] See, Sorell, *supra* note 10 at 9-10. Kraus, *supra* note 1 at 28-29; Huett, *supra* note 118 at 12-19.

[185] Sorell, *supra* note 10 at 9-10.

[186] Ivar Hagendoorn, *The Dancing Brain*, Cerebrum: The Dana Forum on Brain Science, Vol. 5. No. 2, Spring 2003, http://www.ivarhagendoorn.com/files/articles/Hagendoorn-Cerebrum-03.pdf. *Id.*

[187] Sorell, *supra* note 10 at 52.

[188] Lihs, *supra* note 1 at 14.

[189] Kraus, *supra* note 1 at 36. Cynthia Winton-Henry, Dance – The Sacred Art, The Joy of Movement as a Spiritual Practice, (2009) p.2.

[190] Sorell, *supra* note 10 at 19. Sachs, *supra* note 7 at 30, 252; Lihs 14, 17-18.

[191] Lihs, *supra* note 1 at14

[192] See also, Sorell, *supra* note 10 at 19; Sachs, *supra* note 7 at 252.

[193] Isaiah 55:12. *See also*, Cynthia Winton-Henry, *supra* note 189 at 2.

[194] Sorell, *supra* note 10 at 25.

[195] Psalms 149:3. *See also*, Jonas, *supra* note 68 at 38.

[196] Sorell, *supra* note 10 at 19, Sachs, *supra* note 7 at 30 (1 Chr. 15:29; II Samuel, VI:14 - 21).

[197] Sorell, *supra* note 10 at 19

[198] Omid Safi, *What if We Prayed Inside the Ka'aba of the Heart*, On Being.org, June 4, 2015, https://onbeing.org/blog/what-if-we-prayed-inside-the-kaba-of-the-heart/

[199] Sorell, *supra* note 10 at 19-21. Kraus, *supra* note 1. Lihs, *supra* note 1 at 17-19. *See also*, The Hymn of Jesus from the Acts of St. John; The Gnostic Society Library, http://www.gnosis.org/library/hymnjesu.html.

[200] *Id. See also*, Lihs, *supra* note 1 at 17-18.

[201] *Id.* Wosien, *supra* note 2 at 9.

[202] Cynthia Winton-Henry, *supra* note 189 at 3; Lihs, *supra note 1* at 17.

[203] *Id.*

[204] Kraus, *supra* note 1 at 49.

[205] Sorell, *supra* note 10 at 20.

[206] *Id.*

[207] Jonas, *supra* note 68 at 42, Sorell, *supra* note 10 at 36.

[208] Kraus, *supra* note 1 at 55-56, Wagner, Ann Wagner, Adversaries of Dance, From the Puritans to the Present, University of Illinois, 1999. pp. 3-5, Marcelo Gleiser, *supra* note 39 at 64-65; Jonas *supra* note 68 at 44-48, 50.

[209] Peter Michaud, *Image: The Galactic Dance of NGC 5394 and NGC 5395*, phys.org, Dec. 13, 2019, https://phys.org/news/2019-12-image-galactic-ngc.html

[210] Albert Einstein, cited in Peter Michaud supra note 209.

[211] See, Andrew Fraknoi, *How Fast Are You Moving When You are Sitting Still, The Universe in the Classroom*, No. 71, Spr. 2007, https://nightsky.jpl.nasa.gov/docs/HowFast.pdf

[212] Marina Koren, *The Milky Way Could Collide into Another galaxy Billions of Years Earlier than Predicted, Mark Your Calendars for a Rendezvous with the Large Magellanic Cloud*, The Atlantic, Jan. 5, 2019. https://www.theatlantic.com/science/archive/2019/01/cosmic-collision-could-change-milky-way/579520/.

[213] Cynthia Winton-Henry, *supra* note 189 at 8.

[214] *Id.* at 16.

[215] Raguram, R. et al, *Traditional Community Resources for Mental Health: A Report of Temple Healing from India,* British Medical Journal, 2002; 325:38.

[216] Monteiro, *supra* note 156.

[217] Kraus, *supra* note 1 at 23.

[218] Sachs, *supra* note at 7, 41-42.

[219] *Id.* Lihs, *supra* note 1 at 12.

Chapter V

[1] Harvard Health Publishing, *Using Medicine to Tune the Heart*, Newsletter, Aug. 26, 2019. https://www.health.harvard.edu/newsletter_article/using-music-to-tune-the-heart.

[2] *A Pioneer in Motion, Dance Therapy's D.C. Roots*, Wash. Post, pg. Z16, May 5, 1998.

[3] *Id.*

[4] *Id.*

[5] *Id.*

[6] *Id.*

[7] Lisa Delaney, *Dancing Arthritis Away*, Prevention, The Gazette, (Montreal, Quebec), March 22, 1992.

[8] *Id.*

[9] *Id.*

[10] *Id.*

[11] American Dance Therapy Association, https://adta.org/our-mission/.

[12] *Id.*

[13] *Id.*

[14] *Id.*

[15] *Id.*

[16] American Dance Therapy Association, (ADTA) General Questions, https://adta.org/faqs/

[17] *Id.*

[18] Nadja Alexander and Michelle LeBaron, *Dancing to the Rhythm of the Role-Play, Applying Dance Intelligence to Conflict Resolution,* Hamline Journal of Public Law & Policy, 33 Hamline J. Pub. L. & Policy, 327, Spring 2012.

[19] Myrna Davies Washington, *Dance Movement Therapy and Marriage, Couples' and Family Therapy*, 2014, http://www.academia.edu/8092728/Dance_Movement_Therapy_DMT_and_Marriage_Couples_and_Family_Therapies.

[20] Alexander and LeBaron, *supra* note 18. *See,* Howard Gardner's Theory of Multiple Intelligences,

https://www.niu.edu/facdev/_pdf/guide/learning/howard_gardner_theor y_multiple_intelligences.pdf

[21] Koch, S. et al, *Effects of Dance Movement Therapy and Dance on Health-Related Psychological Outcomes: A Meta-Analysis*, The Arts in Psychotherapy, Feb. 2014, vol. 41, Issue 1, pp. 46-64.

[22] Alexander and LeBaron, *supra* note 18.

[23] Roberta Hershenson, *Dance Therapy Beyond Its 'Flower Child' Image*, N.Y. Times, Oct. 15, 1995.

[24] Alexander and LeBaron, *supra* note 18. Jean Nordhaus, Dance as Mental Therapy, Wash. Post, Oct. 8, 1978. Lucy Taylor, *Dance, Manhood and Warfare Amongst the Acholi People of Northern Uganda*, November 28, 2016; https://blogs.loc.gov/kluge/2016/11/dance-manhood-and-warfare-amongst-the-acholi-people-of-northern-uganda/ (Guest Post by Jason Steinhauer).

[25] Id.

[26] *The Kestenberg Movement Profile*, https://www.seas.harvard.edu/climate/eli/KMP/; http://www.kestenbergmovementprofile.org/; ADTA *supra* note 16; Koch *supra* note 21.

[27] ADTA, *supra* notes 11, 16.

[28] Ramona Hanke, *The Impact of Ballroom Dancing on the Marriage Relationships,* Thesis, University of Pretoria, (2006), https://repository.up.ac.za/bitstream/handle/2263/23945/00Dissertation. pdf?sequence=1.

[29] Alexander and LeBaron, *supra* note 18.

[30] *Id.*

[31] *Id.*

[32] Jean Nordhaus, *supra* note 24.

[33] Wagner, https://link.springer.com/article/10.1007/s10465-018-9271-y

[34] Ramona Hanke, *supra* note 28.

[35] *A Pioneer in Motion, supra* note 2.

[36] American Dance Therapy Association, *supra* note 16.

[37] Rachel Schneider, *Dance and Movement Therapy Helpful for Anxiety, Depression*, 13 ABC Action News, Ohio, April 8, 2020, https://www.13abc.com/content/news/Dance--569477781.html

[38] American Dance Therapy Association, *supra* note 16.

[39] *Id.*

[40] *Id.*

[41] Anita Johnson, *Dancing out of Darkness*, Tweed daily News (NSW) Apr. 1, 2015.

[42] Benjamin Tan, *Rhythm for the blues; Dance therapy gives you a good workout and is a fun way to relieve stress*, The Straits Times (Singapore) Nov 13, 2005.

[43] Alexander and LeBaron, *supra* note 18.

[44] *Id.*

[45] *Id.*

[46] *Id.*

[47] Loretta Fong, *Hong Kong Faces, It was a Lonely Journey but the City's First Registered Dance Therapist Has Found Her Reward*, South China Morning Post, Nov. 29, 2007

[48] Alexander and LeBaron, *supra* note 18.

[49] Wagner, https://link.springer.com/article/10.1007/s10465-018-9271-y; Nordhaus, *supra* note 24.

[50] Isabella Pericleous, *Healing Through Movement: Dance/Movement Therapy for major Depression*, Senior Seminar in Dance 2011, (Director: Professor L. Gafarola) Columbia University.

[51] *Id.*

[52] *Id.*

[53] *Id.*

[54] Hugh Wilson, *Creative Therapy Promotes Healing*, Weekend Australian, July 7, 2012.

[55] *Id.*

[56] *Id.*

[57] Sara Keating, *Can Culture Make Us Well*, The Irish Times, May 17, 2008.

[58] *Id.*

[59] *Id.* Bonnie Bainbridge Cohen at https://bonniebainbridgecohen.com/

[60] Thespec.com, *Dance Therapy is Enjoying a Growth Spurt*, December 16, 2013. Katy Daigle, *Healing the Mind by Moving the Body*, The Moscow Times, May 30, 1996.

[61] Zahra Borno, *A Moving Experience: Just A Few Years Ago Alternative Therapies Were Regarded as a Little Bit Cranky. But Experts are Now Coming Around to the Ideas...*" The Bristol Post, Jan. 11, 1999. Hershenson, *supra* note 23. *A Pioneer in Motion*, *supra* note 2.

[62] Katy Daigle, *supra* note 60.

[63] *Id.*

[64] *Id.*

[65] *Id.*

[66] *Id.*

[67] Zhang Xinyuan, *Dance Your Trouble Away*, Global Times (China) Sept. 10, 2014

[68] *Id*

[69] *Id.*

[70] *See,* Steinberg-Oren, S. et al, *Let's Dance: A Holistic Approach to Treating veterans with Posttraumatic Stress Disorder, A Pilot Study Suggested that a Dance Class Program Promoted Wellbeing, Self-Confidence, and Stress Reduction for Veterans with PTSD*, Federal Practice, July 2016; 33(7):44-49. Borno, *supra* note 61. Hershenson, *supra* note 23.

[71] *The Healing Artists; Imagine if your Hospital Team Included a Dancer, a Comic and a Musician…* The Toronto Star, April 2, 2016

[72] *Id.*

[73] *See generally*, Sarah Hampson, *Getting Their Groove Back; From the gym to the ballroom, personal trainer Sarah Robichaud shows Parkinson's patients like Andy Barrie how the tango and waltz can loosen muscles and lift spirits,* The Globe and Mail, Mar. 3, 2008; Gloria Hochman, *Dance Classes Help Parkinson's Patients Stay Limber*, The Philadelphia Inquirer, July 16, 2013; Ese Olumhense, *Parkinson's Disease Progression Can be Slowed with Vigorous Exercise Study Shows*, Chicago Tribune, Dec. 11, 2017.

[74] American Dance Therapy Association, (ADTA) General Questions https://adta.org/faqs/

[75] *Id.*

[76] *Id.*

[77] *Id.*

[78] See generally, India Sturgis, *Could Being a Silver Swan Stop You Ageing?* Irish Daily Mail, March 25, 2015. Delaney, *supra* note 7. *Silver Swan Why Ballet is Great for the Over 50s*, The Sunday Telegraph, (London), Aug. 21, 2016. *Dancing Over the Decades, Professionals and Amateurs both Continue to Enjoy Ballet, Tap and Ballroom at Middle Age and Beyond*, Portland Press Herald (Maine) Jul. 15, 2001.

[79] Karen Weintraub, *Is Art Therapy the Answer for Dementia? Making music, painting, or dancing — and seeing or hearing it — may be the most effective treatment for dementia to date*, The Boston Globe, Nov. 27, 2012.

[80] *Id.*

[81] *Id.*

[82] *Id.*

[83] *Id.*

[84] *Id.*

[85] *Id.*

[86] *Id.*

[87] Tara Bahrampour, *Changing 'the Tragedy Narrative,' Why a Growing Camp is Promoting a More Joyful Approach to Alzheimer's*, Wash. Post, Feb. 21, 2019.

[88] *Id.*

[89] *Id.*

[90] *Id.*

[91] *Id.*

[92] *Id.*

[93] *Id.*

[94] *Id. See* Comments

[95] Sandra Lorenzo, *For Parkinson's Patients, Dancing the Tango Can Help Reconnect Mind and Body*, Huffington Post, Apr. 17, 2015.

[96] *Id.*

[97] *Id.*

[98] *Id.*

[99] *Id.*

[100] *Psychiatric Patients Get Dose of Therapy with Dance Class*, Hamilton Spectator, Ontario, Canada, March 9, 1993.

[101] *Id.*

[102] *Dance therapy helping Parkinson's patients in Ukraine*, Plus Media Solutions (PMS), May 26, 2015.

[103] *See examples such as Rosener House discussed below.*

[104] Kris Kenrick, *A Tango with Alzheimer's, Rosener House first in nation to host French therapeutic dance program*, Palo Alto Weekly, https://www.paloaltoonline.com/news/2019/06/07/a-tango-with-alzheimers;

[105] *Id.*

[106] *Id.*

[107] Maggie Mah, *Positively Determined, Barbara Kalt Wraps Up a Memorable Career but She is Still on a Mission."* The Almanac, June 29, 2019, https://www.almanacnews.com/news/2019/06/29/positively-determined

[108] *Id.*

[109] *Id.*

[110] *Id.*

[111] Kris Kenrick, *supra* note 104.

[112] *Id.*

[113] *Id.*

[114] *Id.*

[115] Maggie Mah, *supra* note 107.

[116] *Id.*

[117] Wu Tao, *The dancing Way, Press, Media Releases & Articles*, https://wutaodance.com/about-us/press/

See also, Anna Brooke, *Healing, Wu Tao Dance*, http://www.annabrookehealing.com/wu-tao-dance

[118] *Id.*

[119] *Id.*

[120] *Id.*

[121] *Id.*

[122] *Id.*

[123] *Id.*

[124] *Id.*

[125] Duignan, D. et al, *Exploring Dance as a Therapy for Symptoms and Social Interaction in a Dementia care Setting*, Nursing Times, July 30, 2009, https://www.nursingtimes.net/roles/mental-health-nurses/exploring-dance-as-a-therapy-for-symptoms-and-social-interaction-in-a-dementia-care-unit-30-07-2009/

[126] *Id.*

[127] *Id.*

[128] Jen Rini, *Dance Therapy for Dementia*, The News Journal, Delaware Online News, Nov. 6, 2016, https://www.delawareonline.com/story/news/health/2016/11/06/dance-therapy-healing-dementia-alzheimers-disease/92724066/

[129] *Id.*

[130] *Id.*

[131] *Id.*

[132] Elizabeth Elizalde and Thomas Tracy, *It's the Little Steps that Count: Dementia Patients Fight Memory Loss by Dancing the Night Away*, N.Y. Daily News, Mar. 2, 2019.

[133] *Id.*

[134] *Id.*

[135] *Id.*

[136] Riverdale Press, Alvin Ailey Dance Foundation, *Ailey Dance Workshop for Caregivers & Individuals with Dementia*, Oct. 16, 2019, https://www.riverdalepress.com/stories/aileydance-workshop-for-caregivers-individuals-with-dementia,70263

[137] *Id.*

[138] *Five Ways Dancing Makes a Difference for those with Dementia*, https://willowtowers.com/5-ways-dancing-makes-a-difference-for-those-with-dementia/.

[139] *Id.*

[140] Natalie Beneviat, *Joy Through Dance Part of Memory Care Program at St. Barnabas*, Hampton Tribune Live, Dec. 16, 2019, https://hampton.triblive.com/joy-through-dance-part-of-memory-care-program-at-st-barnabas/

[141] *Id.*

[142] *Id.*

[143] *Id.*

[144] *Id.*

[145] *Id.*

[146] Rebecca Kitchen, *Dementia Friendly Dance Class Improving Lives*, KOLO 8 News Now, Reno, Jan. 29, 2020, https://www.kolotv.com/content/news/Dementia-Friendly-Dance-Class-Improves-Lives-567390481.html

[147] *Id.*

[148] *Id*

[149] *Id.*

[150] *Id.*

[151] *Id.*

[152] *A Dance Programme Set Up by a Physiotherapist Brings People with Dementia Together,* https://www.alzheimers.org.uk/get-support/publications-and-factsheets/dementia-together-magazine/dance-programme-set-physiotherapist-brings-people-dementia-together

[153] *Id.*

[154] *Id.*

[155] *Id.*

[156] *Id.*

[157] *Id.*

[158] Jonathan Hair, *Dementia and Alzheimer's patients see Symptoms Ease as Dance Brings Clarity and Rejuvenation*, ABC News (Queensland, NSW) https://www.abc.net.au/news/2017-02-17/dementia-and-alzheimers-symptoms-eased-through-dancing/8281508

[159] *Id.*

[160] *Id.*

[161] *Id.*

[162] *Id.*

[163] *Danzon Therapy: Latinos Waltz to Ward off Alzheimer's*, NBC news, Latino, Feb. 3, 2014, https://www.nbcnews.com/news/latino/danzon-therapy-latinos-waltz-ward-alzheimers-n17146

[164] *Id.*

[165] *Id.*

[166] *Id.*

[167] *Id.*

[168] *Id.*

[169] *Id.*

[170] Sarah Taddeo, *How a Landmark UCLA Dementia Program Could Ease Burdens in Rochester Communities of Color*, Democrat & Chronicle, Dec. 20, 2019. https://www.democratandchronicle.com/story/news/2019/12/20/caregivers-color-find-tailored-solutions-ucla-dementia-program-los-angeles-rochester/2638830001/

[171] *Id.*

[172] *Id.*

[173] *Id.*

[174] Almaz Ohene, *Video: Watch Parkinson's Patient Walk Again after Hearing Favorite Song*, Parkinson's Life, 8 February 2017, https://parkinsonslife.eu/video-watch-parkinsons-patient-walk-again-after-hearing-favourite-song/.

[175] Judith Potts, *How Dance Classes Help Sufferers of Parkinson's Disease*, The Telegraph, 13 Aug. 2018, https://www.telegraph.co.uk/health-fitness/body/dance-classes-help-sufferers-parkinsons-disease/.

[176] *Parkinson's Patients Test Irish Set Dancing Benefits*, https://www.bbc.com/news/world-europe-22066905.

[177] Ese Olumhense, *supra* note 73.

[178] Lauren Moss, *Dance to Prevent Decline: Dementia, Parkinson's*, WNDU News, June 11, 2019, https://www.wndu.com/content/news/Dance-to-prevent-decline-Dementia-and-Parkinsons-511141321.html

[179] *Id.*

[180] *Id.*

[181] Ruth A. Richter, A New Rhythm, Dance Benefits Parkinson's Patients, Stanford Medicine, Winter 2017, http://stanmed.stanford.edu/2017winter/dance-for-parkinsons-disease-at-the-stanford-neuroscience-health-center.html.

[182] *Id.*

[183] *Id.*

[184] *Id.*

[185] Gail Kent, *Parkinson's Patients Learn to Go with Dance Flow at Two Left Feet*, The Virginian-Pilot, Aug. 11, 2019, https://www.pilotonline.com/entertainment/arts/article_5fd29c76-b7cc-11e9-bf5c-03bb96a165be.html

[186] *Id.*

[187] *Id.*

[188] Anne Gehris, *A New Rhythm for Parkinson's: Dance Classes Alleviate Symptoms, Conscious Effort to Learn Moves helps Rebuild Bridge Between Body and Brain*, The Gazette, Montreal, Nov. 15, 2005.

[189] Lou Francher, *Parkinson's Disease Patients Find Rare Physical Freedom in Berkeley Based Dance Classes*, San Jose Mercury News, June 22, 2011.

[190] *Id.*

[191] Richter, *supra* note 181.

[192] *Id.*

[193] *Id.*

[194] *Id.*

[195] Victor Swoboda, *Parkinson's Disease Doesn't Slow Down this Dance Group*, The Gazette (Montreal) Oct. 2, 2013.

[196] *Id.*

[197] Annette Dasey, *Dance: The New Parkinson's Remedy Ageing Well*, Sunday Telegraph, Feb. 16, 2016.

[198] *Id.*

[199] Gail Kent, *Parkinson's Patients Learn to Go with Dance Flow at Two Left Feet*, The Virginian-Pilot, Aug. 11, 2019, https://www.pilotonline.com/entertainment/arts/article_5fd29c76-b7cc-11e9-bf5c-03bb96a165be.html

[200] *Id.*

[201] *Id.*

[202] *Id.*

[203] *Id.*

[204] *Id.*

[205] *Id.*

[206] *Id.*

[207] *Id.*

[208] *Id.*

[209] *Id.*

[210] *Id.*

[211] *Id.*

[212] *Id.*

[213] Richter *supra* note 181.

[214] *Id.*

[215] *Id.*

[216] *Id.*

[217] *Id.*

[218] *Id.*

[219] *Id.*

[220] Beth Reese Cravey, *'Everybody has the right to dance'; JU offers dance class for Parkinson's patients*, Florida Times-Union (Jacksonville) Aug. 13, 2017.

[221] Sandra Lorenzo, *supra* note 95.

[222] *Id.*

[223] Andrea Zani, *Moving with a Mission, Weekly Zumba Class Helps Parkinson's Sufferers Keep their Muscles and memories Sharp*, Wisconsin State Journal, June 26, 2011; See also, *Autism, Arthritis, Parkinson's... is there anything ZUMBA can't tackle?* Irish Daily Mail, October 8, 2013.

[224] Carol Krucoff, *Before the Fall, Dancing, Strength Training and Other Exercises May Stem the Rise in Senior's Injuries*, Wash. Post, July 25, 2000.

[225] Sally Bowell and Sally Marie Bamford, *A Report from the Commission on Dementia and Music (2018), The International Longevity Centre*, https://ilcuk.org.uk/wp-content/uploads/2018/10/Commission-on-Dementia-and-Music-report.pdf

[226] Karen Weintraub, *supra* note 79.

[227] *Id.*

[228] *Id.*

[229] *Id.*

[230] *Id.*

[231] *Id.*

[232] Hearthstone Alzheimer Care, Family Feedback, https://www.thehearth.org/about/family-feedback/

[233] *Id.*

[234] Jen Hayward, Comment, in Karen Weintraub, *supra* note 79.

[235] See, Sally Bowell and Sally Marie Bamford supra note 687; Tara Bahrampour, *Behavioral Therapies Better than Antipsychotics for Dementia Patients, Nurses Say*, Wash. Post, Mar. 17, 2014. Tara Bahrampour, *Seniors with Dementia, Express themselves, Connect with Others in Drumming Circle*, Wash. Post, June 19, 2013. Karen Weintraub, *supra* note 79.

[236] Weintraub, *supra* note 79.

[237] *Id.*

[238] Laura Donnelly, *Dementia Patients should be Offered Music and Dance Therapy*, The Telegraph, https://www.telegraph.co.uk/news/2019/04/05/dementia-patients-should-offered-music-dance-therapy/. Tara Bahrampour, *Behavioral Therapies* supra note 235.

[239] *Id.*

[240] Sofia Rizzi, *Music and dance therapy should be offered to dementia patients*, research shows, https://www.classicfm.com/discover-music/music-and-dance-therapy-dementia/

[241] Jonathan Graff-Radford, *How Can Music Help people who Have Alzheimer's Disease? Mayo Clinic*,

https://www.mayoclinic.org/diseases-conditions/alzheimers-disease/expert-answers/music-and-alzheimers/faq-20058173

[242] *Id.*

[243] *Id.*

[244] *Id.*

[245] Michelle Kelley, *The Benefits of Silent Dance Therapy for People with Dementia*, June 11, 2018, https://www.cottageassistedliving.com/blog/the-benefits-of-silent-dance-therapy-for-people-with-dementia/

[246] *Id.*

[247] *Id.*

[248] *Moove and Groove, Our Story*, https://www.mooveandgroove.com.au/about-us/

[249] Sarah Hampson, *supra* note 73.

[250] *Id.*

[251] *Id.*

[252] Gloria Hochman, supra note 73.

[253] *Id.*

[254] Beth Reese Cravey, *supra* note 220.

[255] See e.g. Anna Medaris Miller, *What is Ecstatic Dance – and Can it Improve Your Health? The Ancient, Inherent Practice is Gaining Modern Appeal*, US News & World Report, May 24, 2018, https://health.usnews.com/wellness/articles/2018-05-24/what-is-ecstatic-dance-and-can-it-improve-your-health.

[256] Harvard Health Publishing, *Using Medicine to Tune the Heart*, *supra* note 1.

[257] Borno, *supra* note 61. Hershenson, *supra* note 23.

[258] Harvard Health Publishing, *Using Medicine to Tune the Heart*, *supra* note 1.

[259] *Id.*

[260] *Dance Therapy Cures Tedium,* Maroochy Weekly (Queensland), Dec 6, 2012.

[261] Eyre, Harris A et al, *Changes in Neural Connectivity and Memory Following a Yoga Intervention for Older Adults: A Pilot Study,"* *Journal of Alzheimer's disease : JAD* vol. 52,2 (2016): 673-84. doi:10.3233/JAD-150653.

[262] Amanda MacMillan, Yoga is Officially Sweeping the Workplace, Jan 5, 2017

Alison Coleman, Is Google's Model of the Creative Workplace the Future of the Office, The Guardian, 11 Feb 2016, https://www.theguardian.com/careers/2016/feb/11/is-googles-model-of-the-creative-workplace-the-future-of-the-office.

[263] Erik Hogstrom, *Getting Jiggy, Burn Calories While Showing Some Moves on the Dance Floor*, Telegraph Herald, (Dubuque Iowa) Feb. 14, 2005.

[264] *A Move for a Move*, My Republica (Nepal), April 11, 2014.

[265] Heena Khhandelwal and Pratik Ghosh, Yoga with a Twist, DNA, April 16, 2017.

[266] *Id.*

[267] *Id.*

[268] *Id.*

[269] *Id.*

[270] *'Dance Therapy Reduces Stress, Boosts Self-esteem'*, The Pioneer, Oct. 3, 2012.

[271] *Bharatanatyam with Benefits,* Times of India, Feb. 28, 2016.

[272] *Id.*

[273] *Id.*

[274] *Id.*

[275] Shita Sengupta, *World Dance Day, How dance Rejuvenates Your Mind and Body*, Indian Express, April 29, 2017.

[276] Dance Your Way to Good Health, New India Express, June 18, 2013.

[277] *Id.*

[278] Shita Sengupta, supra note 275.

[279] *Finding Fitness Through Dance*, New India Express, Sept. 20, 2014.

[280] *Id.*

[281] *Dance Your Way to Good Health, supra* note 276. 'To relieve stress, opt for dance therapy' The Pioneer, India, Jan. 17, 2011.

[282] *Id.*

[283] Bharatanatyam with benefits, *supra* note 271.

[284] *Id.*

[285] *'Dance therapy Reduces Stress, Boosts Self-esteem', supra* note 270.

[286] Anna Medaris Miller, *supra* note 255.

[287] *Id.*

[288] *Id.*

[289] *Id.*

[290] Comment of Tam Hunt, (May 3, 2019) in Marilyn Friedman, *Is Dancing the Kale of Exercise, Research Shows that Dance Offers a Wealth of Anti-Aging Benefits. It's also Fun*, N.Y. Times, April 30, 2019.

[291] Sinead Hickie, Fit Tips, Sunday Tribune (Ireland) Sept. 22, 2002. Retrieved from https://advance.lexis.com/api/document?collection=news&id=urn:contentItem:470M-6BY0-015B-G12H-00000-00&context=1516831. SynergyDance.com, https://synergydance.com/#about.

[292] *Id.*

[293] *Healing workshop with author Marsha Scarbrough*, Las Cruces Sun-News, Mar. 11, 2009.
Marsha Scarbrough, http://www.marshascarbrough.com/events.htm.
[294] *Id.*

[295] Jane Alexander, *Exploring Alternatives…The Fairbane Method*, The Express, Feb. 21, 2000.
[296] *Id.*

[297] Joanna Hunter, *Go On, Give Us a Hug*, The Times (London), Aug. 28, 2004.
[298] *Id.*

[299] Sarah Taylor, *Biodanza: Moves to Shape your Body and Min*d, Pretoria News, April 2, 2011, E1 Edition.
[300] *Id.*

[301] *Id.*

[302] *Id.*

[303] Kathrin Rehfeld et al; Dancing or Fitness Sport? *The Effect of Two Training Programs on Hippocampal Plasticity and Balance Ability*, Frontiers in Human Neuroscience, Front. Hum. Neurosci., 15 June 2017 | https://doi.org/10.3389/fnhum.2017.00305; https://www.frontiersin.org/articles/10.3389/fnhum.2017.00305/full. Science Daily, "Dancing Can Reverse the Signs of Aging in the Brain, https://www.sciencedaily.com/releases/2017/08/170825124902.htm, August 25, 2017
[304] *Id.*

[305] Anna Medaris Miller, When Night Clubs Meets Fitness Studios, Dance Parties are Popping Up at Gym and Fitness Centers Globally, US News & World Report, Jan 5, 2015, https://health.usnews.com/health-news/health-wellness/articles/2015/01/05/when-night-clubs-meet-fitness-studios.
[306] *Id.*

[307] *Id.*

[308] Lauren Steussy, *Picture Diary Places first at Autism App Jam*, Orange County Register, May 1, 2014.
[309] *Id.*

Chapter VI

[1] *See*, Jem Spectar, We Dance for Light, Complementary Medicine for Depression and Anxiety in the Age of Angst, *(forthcoming)*. See also, Jem Spectar, Rx MED: Preventive Medicine for Heart Disease, Cancer and Diabetes & Healthy Aging *(forthcoming)*.

[2] Trish Vella-Burrows and Lian Wilson, *Remember to Dance, Evaluating the Impact of Dance Activities for People in Different Stages of Dementia*, Sidney De Haan Research Centre for Arts and Health, p. 12, https://www.greencandledance.com/wp-content/uploads/2014/02/141-KC-15-SDH_DanceDementia_Report-2016-proof-08.pdf.

[3] Lee, I. et al, *Association of Step Volume and Intensity with All-Cause Mortality in Older Women. JAMA Intern. Med.* 2019;179(8):1105–1112. doi:10.1001/jamainternmed.2019.0899.

[4] *Id. See also*, Shari Roan, *Women Should Exercise an Hour a Day to Maintain Weight, Study Says,* LA Times, March 24, 2010, https://www.latimes.com/archives/la-xpm-2010-mar-24-la-sci-women-weight-gain24-2010mar24-story.html

[5] Duck Chul Lee et al, *Leisure-Time Running Reduces All-Cause and Cardiovascular Mortality Risk,* Journal of the American College of Cardiology, 2014; 64 (5): 472 DOI: 10.1016/j.jacc.2014.04.058. *See also*, Christie Aschwanden, *The Longevity Files, A Strong Grip? Push-ups? What Actually Can Help You Live to a Ripe Old Age?* Wash. Post, Sept. 28, 2019, https://www.washingtonpost.com/health/the-longevity-files-a-strong-grip-pushups-what-actually-can-help-you-live-to-a-ripe-old-age/2019/09/27/e2cffb5c-da34-11e9-ac63-3016711543fe_story.html

[6] Lisa Delaney et al, *Dancing Arthritis Away, Prevention Magazine*, The Gazette, (Montreal, Quebec), March 22, 1992.)

[7] As Einstein, stated: "Everything is determined by forces over which we have no control... Human beings, vegetables, or cosmic dust, we all dance to a mysterious tune, intoned in the distance by an invisible piper."